HOUSE OFFICER
Becoming a Medical Specialist

HOUSE OFFICER
Becoming a Medical Specialist

Richard L. Cohen, M.D.

University of Pittsburgh School of Medicine
Pittsburgh, Pennsylvania

Plenum Medical Book Company • New York and London

Library of Congress Cataloging in Publication Data

Cohen, Richard L. (Richard Lawrence), 1922-
  House officer: becoming a medical specialist / Richard L. Cohen.
      p.   cm.
  Includes bibliographies and index.
  ISBN 0-306-42942-X
  1. Medicine—Specialties and specialists—United States. I.. Title.
  [DNLM: 1. Education, Medical, Graduate—United States. 2. Internship and Residen-
cy. 3. Specialties, Medical—United States. W 20 C678h]
  R729.5.S6C64   1988
  610'.7'1173—dc19
  DNLM/DLC   88-17930
  for Library of Congress   CIP

© 1988 Plenum Publishing Corporation
233 Spring Street, New York, N.Y. 10013

Plenum Medical Book Company is an imprint of Plenum Publishing Corporation

Printed in the United States of America

ACKNOWLEDGMENTS

The task of thanking everyone who made a contribution to a volume of this type is a large though pleasant one. Without question, the greatest debt of gratitude is owed to the 52 very busy, often very tired interns and residents who gave their valuable time to be interviewed. Even more importantly, they shared their thoughts and feelings to a degree I could not have predicted. Without their contribution, this book would not exist.

Dr. Thomas Detre not only encouraged me to pursue this work, but through his good offices, encouraged many senior department chairmen and training directors to cooperate in its implementation. He has provided thoughtful counsel both during the period of information collection and, later, during my struggles to get all of this on paper in readable form.

Thanks also go, of course, to all of the faculty members, chief residents, and training directors who helped interpret this work to sometimes skeptical groups of house officers in their departments and who, undoubtedly, were responsible for the unpredictably large number of volunteers.

Several full-time hospital physicians and private practitioners were kind enough to read many of these interviews and to provide helpful comments. Among these were Drs. Lee Bass, Peter Henderson, Joseph Horton, Jonas Johnson, Michael Rancurello, James Reilly, Paul Scott, Arnold Sladen, and Barry Uretsky. Maggie McDonald and Barbara Epstein also provided suggestions and encouragement.

My secretary Karen Hickey-Rhinaman provided continuity of care during the entire process, doggedly tracking down elusive house officers, scheduling and rescheduling broken appointments, transcribing taped interviews, and finally, paying close attention to the production of the manuscript.

Last but not least, my deepest appreciation goes to Janice Stern, my editor at Plenum, who proved to be an author's dream, smoothing a furrowed brow here and providing an encouraging shove there, all the while making sure the writer's self-esteem did not sag below the critical level that would interfere with productivity.

My apologies to anyone I have neglected. As any reader can see, this not overly long work required the efforts of a great many people.

R.L.C.

A NOTE TO THE READER

This book contains many quotations from interviews with interns and residents, and there are frequent transitions from text to quoted material. In order to assist the reader with these transitions, upright and inverted triangles have been employed.

A Glossary has been included at the end of the book for the non-medical reader.

CONTENTS

IV. THE "GENERAL" SPECIALTIES

V. GENERIC ISSUES

VI. CONCLUSIONS AND RECOMMENDATIONS

Chapter 1

INTRODUCTION

This book is about how young physicians experience training as medical specialists. Much attention is now being drawn to the stresses of postgraduate medical education, their potential negative impact on the quality of patient care, and the manner in which these stresses influence the professional and personal development of the physicians involved.

The entire focus of this book is on the firsthand experience of 52 such physicians enrolled in 16 different medical specialty training programs. Because the evaluation of stress is largely a subjective one, I have elected to approach the question through the perception and the cognitive processes of the trainees themselves.

THE DOCTORS

The "subjects" of this work are 52 young physicians who volunteered to be interviewed confidentially and anonymously during the 1986–1987 academic year. They represent the specialties of anesthesiology, clinical pathology, dermatology, emergency medicine, family practice, general surgery, internal medicine, neurology, neurosurgery, obstetrics and gynecology, ophthalmology, orthopedic surgery, otolaryngology, pediatrics, psychiatry, and radiology.

Because this inquiry depended entirely on a volunteer sample, it was not possible to ensure a wholly representative population. For instance, not a single minority house officer stepped forward. The actual demographic breakdown is represented in Table 1. Although all of the subjects did not come from the same training center, an effort was made to compare the characteristics of this population with that of a large, metropolitan, university-affiliated medical center. The demographics of that population are represented in Table 2. As can be seen, there are several discrepancies, although most segments of the population are well represented, with the exception of minority groups.

METHOD

I recruited volunteers by approaching their training directors and their service chiefs, explaining the specific purpose of the project, and requesting permission to contact the house officer group in that specialty to solicit participants. Because legal and ethical consultation reinforced my judgment that this was not a research project, formal informed consent was not a part of the procedure. Nevertheless, the project was carefully explained to each resident group, and the right to withdraw at any time was made explicit, along with a full guarantee of anonymity. The residents were assured that either the results of this work would be reported in the aggregate, or if specific illustrations were used, the identity of the individual would be thoroughly disguised. This assurance also

TABLE 1
Characteristics of House Officers*

	Medical[a] (18)	Surgical[b] (18)	Hospital-based[c] (9)	General specialists[d] (7)	Total N	%
Gender	M = 11	M = 17	M = 7	M = 7	42	80.8
	F = 7	F = 1	F = 2	F = 0	10	19.2
Age	<25 = 1	<25 = 0	<25 = 0	<25 = 0	1	1.9
	25–29 = 14	25–29 = 11	25–29 = 7	25–29 = 7	39	75.0
	30–35 = 2	30–35 = 6	30–35 = 2	30–35 = 0	10	19.2
	>35 = 1	>35 = 1	>35 = 0	>35 = 0	2	3.9
Race	W = 18	W = 18	W = 9	W = 7	52	100.0
	B = 0	B = 0	B = 0	B = 0	0	0.0
	0 = 0	0 = 0	0 = 0	0 = 0	0	0.0
Marital	M = 8	M = 11	M = 8	M = 3	30	57.7
status	S = 9	S = 6	S = 1	S = 2	18	34.6
	D = 0	D = 1	D = 0	D = 0	1	1.9
	0 = 1	0 = 0	0 = 0	0 = 2	3	5.8
Children	6	7	4	4	21	40.4
Postgraduate	I = 3	I = 2	I = 1	I = 0	6	11.5
year of	II = 9	II = 5	II = 2	II = 5	21	40.4
training	III = 6	III = 6	III = 4	III = 2	18	34.6
	IV = 0	IV = 0	IV = 2		2	3.9
	V = 0	V = 4			4	7.7
		VI = 1			1	1.9

*N = 52. Key: M, male; F, female; >, greater than; <, less than; M, married; S, single; D, divorced; O, other; W, white; B, black; O, other. [a]Internal medicine, pediatrics, psychiatry, neurology, and dermatology. [b]General surgery, obstetrics and gynecology, orthopedic surgery, otolaryngology, ophthalmology, and neurosurgery. [c]Radiology, clinical pathology, and anesthesiology. [d]Emergency medicine and family practice.

served the purpose of allowing the fullest possible freedom to express a range of views about training and about the faculty without concern about later penalties.

In many instances, the service chief or the senior resident in the specialty offered to recruit participants himself or herself, expressing enthusiasm about the work and the desirability of eliciting this information. Only limitations on my own time controlled the size of the sample. More volunteers than I could adequately interview were available in several of the specialties.

As a result of my own experience in counseling residents about either personal difficulties or career choices over the past 35 years, and in the hope of collecting reasonably uniform data, I designed a semistructured interview that I followed in all instances. The interview format was typed and photocopied and explained to each resident at the beginning of the interview so that he or she could more fully participate and so that there would not be any future surprises. This outline appears in the appendix at the end of this chapter.

All interviews were tape-recorded with the explicit permission of the resident. The tape recorder was placed in full view and was not turned on until the resident concurred. The approach of the interview was fundamentally developmental. It reviewed the resident's current assignments

TABLE 2
1986–1987 Statistics*

Number of university residents (555)	Totals	Percentages
Gender	M = 406	73.0
	F = 149	27.0
Age	<25 = 7	1.3
	25–29 = 342	61.6
	30–35 = 161	29.0
	>35 = 45	8.1
Race	W = 524	94.4
	B = 13	2.3
	0 = 18	3.2
Marital status	Approximately one half were married.	

*Key: M, male; F, female; W, white; B, black; O, other.

and work schedule, his or her typical day at the current time, and on-call procedures. Then, it turned to the recent past and covered matters such as career choice, selection of this particular program for training, and similar matters. It then covered more remote subjects, such as preparation in medical school or earlier for the selection of medicine and this specialty as experienced through contacts with others and through early life influences. It then looked at current physical and emotional support systems, stress-coping mechanisms and the resident's own thoughts about those stresses that were inherent in the program and those that might be ameliorated by modifications in the training. The interview paid particular attention to the assets and liabilities perceived in the attending staff and faculty; considered future projects and plans, particularly as they were being shaped by current experiences; and provided space for the resident to introduce other matters as he or she felt they were pertinent. All of this material was covered in approximately one hour. This was possible because, in almost all instances, the resident knew what the structure of the interview was to be and what its goals were and was fully participating. Considerable discipline on the part of the interviewer was a necessary ingredient, however. All of these trainees presented excellent opportunities for exploring other avenues. Many tidbits of information were held out that could easily have seduced the interviewer into tangential areas that would undoubtedly have been curiosity-gratifying but that also would have diffused the pursuit of the primary goal.

I attempted several trial runs of the interview with residents within my own department, found it comfortable both for them and for myself, and was pleased to learn that I could rather easily fit it into one hour. No notes were taken because of the tape recorder. Extensive notes were taken later when the tape was replayed.

The semistructured interview permitted a kind of collation of the ideas, impressions, and recommendations both of the house officers and of myself, which appear in the body of this book. It is important to underscore that this study was not represented to them, nor is it represented to the reader, as a scientific study. Its only value lies in the breadth (16 specialties) of its scope and the semistructured look (brief though it may be) at the developmental status of more than 50 house officers and at the collation of their collective thinking about their training and its assets and liabilities in the late 1980s.

I was at first discouraged by my colleagues from attempting this effort because I was told that I could not get this many house officers in specialties unrelated to psychiatry to speak freely with a psychiatrist. In fact, there was no difficulty at all in this area. There were volunteers in every department. These were not individuals seeking help through the back door. Most were strong, accomplished, and highly competent young men and women adapting very well to the demands of their training. Other faculty colleagues assured me that there would be no volunteers unless I offered reimbursement. In fact, a large number of house officers thanked me for the opportunity to express themselves clearly and in an organized way to a senior faculty member. No payment was offered or requested in any instance.

Other "payments" were extracted from me, however. It is not possible to look at the stresses of training without becoming involved in them. Because of the exigencies of their schedules, I often found myself interviewing residents at very odd times and in unusual places. Although it was often possible to schedule interviews in my office, many were carried out, with frequent interruptions, in nursing stations, doctors' dressing rooms in surgical suites, staff cafeterias, medical record rooms, and, in one instance, on the front seat of an emergency vehicle.

THE APPROACH

As I attempted later to organize and assemble the information derived from these interviews in the preparation of this book, it became clear that some issues were generic to postgraduate medical training and that some seemed more specialty-based. Therefore, the body of this work is broken down into those two general areas. First, we look at issues that seem to be more germane to a given specialty (even these are clustered under medical, surgical, and hospital-based specialties and the group I have labeled the "general specialties"). We then look at what appear to be common themes or threads that run through many, if not most, of the stories that are recounted. These have more to do with such concerns as the content of training, its usefulness in preparation for the future, the attention given by the attending staff, the stresses of fatigue and sleep deprivation, financial and family concerns, incursions into social life, and the pursuit of avocations.

Finally, there is a presentation of conclusions and some recommendations that I believe can be derived from these contacts. In my opinion, although they are not totally substantiated by the data, they are worthy of serious thought from both professionals and lay people. They suggest the existence of problems that go beyond single-minded concerns about physical fatigue and sleep deprivation. In fact, I believe they bear on the philosophy and substance of postgraduate medical education as it is now being conducted in the United States.

Although the reader will not find sections within this book that involve formal interviews with faculty members and attending physicians, I did take the opportunity to have many of the interviews read by specialists in each field. Many did not express surprise at the content; felt that, in general, the interviews reflected an accurate picture of the rewards and problems of training at this time; and believed that the residents, on the whole, had been fair and reasonable in their portrayal of their daily experiences.

LIMITATIONS

Nevertheless, I am mindful that this work does indeed represent the situation almost entirely from the point of view of the trainee. In that sense, it cannot pretend to be balanced or objective. Furthermore, the trainees were located in one urban area (although they came from all parts of the United States), and they were all Caucasian. Undoubtedly, interviews with resident groups containing a higher representation of the minorities would reveal other stresses and yet other coping mechanisms. I had neither the power nor the inclination to commandeer "volunteers." This would have skewed the findings so as to make them even less reliable.

APPENDIX: FLOW OF SEMISTRUCTURED
INTERVIEW WITH HOUSE OFFICERS

I. Explanation of interview format and discussion of purpose of interview

II. Demographic information (age, educational background, hometown, marital status, etc.)

III. Current training situation, for example:

A. Level in specialty or subspecialty
B. Current assignment or rotation

C. "Typical" day, exploring rewards and demands of stress and how these are handled—interactions with peer group, faculty, staff, medical students, etc.

IV. Factors influencing specialty choice

    A. Past
    B. Current

 V. Factors influencing choice of medicine as a career

    A. Personal and motivational
    B. Interpersonal and educational

VI. Review of present situation, including rewards and interests outside of training; trade-offs in time, energy, and finances involved in career pursuits; and hoped-for rewards to come

Part I

THE "MEDICAL" SPECIALTIES

This is the first of four sections in which we will be hearing in detail from a large number of house officers about their work, their education, their plans for the future, and, most specifically, about the daily pains and pleasures attendant to pursuing their careers as specialists. Although, to some degree, I have divided these specialties arbitrarily, the reasons for my having done so may also emerge as these young people speak about their choices, their learning styles, their turn-ons and turn-offs, and their ways of coping with stress.

In this first group, we consider five kinds of trainees, known generally as the *medical specialties*: internal medicine, pediatrics, psychiatry, neurology, and dermatology.

It will become obvious as we proceed through these specialties, that the development of high-technology, invasive diagnostic procedures has made the medical specialist more of an "operator," just as the development of surgical intensive-care units has forced surgeons to become more "intensively" involved in the ongoing medical care of their patients.

We need to remind ourselves that the so-called physician and surgeon really have very different origins. The historical roots of the physician lie in the herbalists, the healers by potion, by poultice, and by tincture. Surgeons trace their own roots back to the thousands of barber-surgeons who emerged all over Europe during ancient and medieval times, and who, by their deft use of the blade, were able to remove warts, tumors, deformities, and other growths. Today, we see the heritage of these differences, as many a school of medicine is still referred to as the *College of Physicians and Surgeons*.

Although I have been licensed as a doctor of medicine for more than 35 years, I have never looked closely at the licenses I have received from three states. They all refer to my authorization to practice as a "physician and surgeon." Obviously, the distinction between these two broad groups of practitioners has existed for centuries and was not something created by the overspecialization of modern medicine.

Chapter 2

INTERNAL MEDICINE

Dr. S. is a 27-year-old second-year resident in internal medicine. He is engaged to be married to a young woman who is currently working for an M.B.A. at the same university in Ohio where Dr. S. attended medical school. They plan to be reunited and to be married in about 18 months, when they simultaneously completed their respective educational obligations. At present, they are able to see each other only about once a month. Dr. S. appeared several minutes early for his interview. He is all angles, rangy, with very long limbs. As he unwound himself from the chair to meet me, I was struck by the gawky Ichabod Crane quality of his gait and posture. His white lab coat covered a uniform consisting of the bright green top of a surgical scrub suit and black wool slacks. His pockets were stuffed with 4×6 index cards, pens, a small loose-leaf notebook, a stethoscope, an ophthalmoscope, a reflex hammer and a tuning fork. About 15 minutes into our interview, his pager began to beep. Without responding, he reached to his belt and turned it off, adding that he had signed out to another resident and they had no business calling him now.

▼   ▼   ▼

My present assignment is on one of the general medical inpatient floors. This is the key year of the residency because of this kind of rotation. You're in immediate charge of the floor. You have three medical interns assigned to you. There are about 30 patients, so they each have about 10 and you're supposed to kind of oversee the whole process. You grow up pretty fast when you have three green interns looking to you for direction all the time.

Actually, it's not entirely like that because we have so many levels of attendings in this department. Someone is always looking over your shoulder. For those patients who are private, their own doctor calls the shots. We can discuss things with him, but if he wants them done a certain way, he gets the last word. Once in a while, an attending does something you may really object to. Some residents will try to buck that.

I remember last year it was obvious that a patient was being brought in mostly as a a control subject for a study that was being done. There was no clinical justification for all the tests that were ordered. The patient's entire hospitalization was not indicated. We were wasting his time and ours. I was just the intern on the case. I knew better than to shoot my mouth off. My resident protested, and there was a lot of flak over it. In the end, the attending had his way.

For us, what separates the good attendings from the bad ones is not that kind of stuff so much. Those incidents are pretty uncommon. It's their investment in teaching and the quality of teaching they do. Generally, there is a real difference between the private attendings and the university faculty. The private guys don't make too much of an effort to teach. They're in too much of a hurry to get out and get back to their offices.

Even among the full-time faculty, there's enormous variation. Some are just natural teachers and have a big investment. Others can't communicate well and don't seem to care about it much. I suppose they were recruited to do research. They just tell you what they want done without explaining things or discussing them with you. You don't learn from those people. I guess they feel their immediate problem is what to do with this patient and not your training. And of course, there's nothing in their training or ours that teaches you how to teach.

I'll probably be in their position some day. I don't know how to teach and no one will show me. I'll either be good or bad at it, and I won't know what the med students and house officers are saying behind my back. It's good to have researchers in the department because they bring in a lot of grant money and are a feather in the department's cap, but for the residents, you have to have the other people, too. Some of the researchers have become so superspecialized that they seem to have forgotten the rest of medicine. They're not just uninterested in teaching; they don't have very much to teach anymore. And especially at the beginning of your internship or residency, you badly need that kind of help.

In some departments, no faculty are asked to do attending rounds unless the residents want them. It's considered an honor. In this department, it's assigned as a chore, and lots of attendings don't like to do it. The residents do have a little feedback checklist that we fill out after each assignment and also to show who we would prefer as attendings, but I'm not convinced that anybody reads it or that it has any effect on future assignments. It's just parceled out as an unpleasant assignment that people have to do. I think good teachers are born, not made. There are good teachers and bad teachers and the department chairman ought to keep the bad teachers away from the residents.

The way the system works now, we do rounds on the same patients three or four times a day. Between four and five hours get invested in this, and I'm not at all sure how necessary it is. The first rounding of the day is without an attending. I do it, starting at about 7:45 A.M. on all 30 patients with the three interns, in about 45 minutes. We stop outside each room, and if there is nothing special that's new or they don't have any problems, we just keep on moving. We spend a little time with the patients where there has been some problem during the night or there are new lab findings. Some residents walk into every room and chat with the patient. I find that drags things out too much. I'm only interested in what problems have developed.

Then I'm off to morning report, where the residents in charge of each ward go over new admissions or any special things they want help with. Often, the chairman is there along with the most senior section chiefs. This is the second time you've gone over the patients. It takes about an hour.

After that, you return to the ward, and it's time for rounds with the attending who's assigned to the floor. You are there, but the interns report. So this is the third rounding and it kills the rest of the morning. Later on, the private attending may come in and want to go over any patients he or she has on the floor. You can't imagine the time that goes into this. Sometimes, I feel a little silly saying that I'm in charge of the floor. After all those people have had their say, you can imagine how much input I have. Often, I feel like a fifth wheel.

Then, in the afternoon, the new admissions start hitting the floor. There are often three or four. Both the interns and I have to work them up. They spend much more time at it. They have to do a very complete history and physical, draw the bloods for the lab, and write very extensive notes. I only spend about 20 to 30 minutes with each patient...but along with my handling problems on the floor, the telephone, writing my own notes, and keeping an eye on the interns, the afternoon and a good part of the evening are gone.

The hours are horrendous, the pay is not very good, and the expectations of the attendings are extremely high. All you can really get out of this is the opportunity to use what you've learned and to make decisions about patient care and to see what works and what doesn't work. In many ways, I think I have developed much more on my rotations at the VA Hospital than on the University assignments. At the VA, it's a more classical experience, where there are no real attendings and you do make most of the decisions. I learned a lot more there than I have at the University Hospital.

The VA environment is what I thrive on. It's really the only reward you have in this second year: the ability to make decisions and see the results of them. This residency has a lot of pluses, but it's kind of short on developing your clinical judgment except at the VA.

Once a week, we have what's called continuity clinic, where you get to follow your own patients over time. It's good because the wards don't allow you to have that kind of long-term contact. The problem is they don't allow any time for it. On the afternoon you have your clinic, you still have to go up to the ward when you're finished and start working up your new admis-

sions. On those days, you're lucky to be out by 11 P.M. If you happen also to
be on night float that night, you're putting in a continuous 36-hour day with
no breaks. It's a crazy system. The floor people want you up there, and the
clinic people want you there, and everybody's angry with you...and you're
in a state of exhaustion. Your judgment goes down the tubes. When I listen
to morning report, I hear many more mistakes being made by the person
who's on night float than by anybody else.

Another experience during this year that's important but a real drain on
you is the ER. I've done that already, but it sure stays with you. Part of the
time you're on days and part nights...like 6 P.M. to 8 A.M. It's very chain
yanking on your physiology. You feel like you've got jet lag a good part
of the time.

At night, in addition to serious emergencies that are always coming in,
there is a steady stream of street people seeking either shelter or drugs...or
both. Also, families bringing in their old folks whom they don't want to take
care of...or can't. They want them admitted to the hospital for some minor
thing, and they don't want to hear that these people don't have diseases that
warrant admissions to an acute-care tertiary hospital. Or private patients
walk in with minor complaints, and you are faced with calling private attendings at 3 A.M. If you call them, they are sore; if you don't call them, they are
sore. One thing I've learned is that lots of private attendings keep the phone
on the side of the bed where their spouse sleeps; that way you can wake
them both up.

When you're faced with people coming into the ER in the middle of the
night with sore throats or back pain, they don't even get good care. You are
trying to deal with them in the wrong setting. At first, I was in a rage at
people coming in in the middle of the night with minor, long-standing complaints. Now, I've gotten used to it, and I have a standard routine I go
through with them in order to get them through and get them out. I remember last year, I had a third-year medical student come in at 5 A.M. with a bad
cold. I asked him what he wanted from me and what he had been told about
what we do for colds. He told me, so I asked him if he already knew, what he
wanted me to do. That was one of the times I really lost my cool. I prac-
tically threw him out. After a while, you don't get angry anymore; you just
get numb.

I remember another guy who came in about 3 A.M. who had already
been seen by the surgical resident for some reason. He had a million different
physical complaints. He said he had scabies and he had all these little 'in-
sects' stuck on Scotch tape to show the doctor. He also complained of chest
pain. The resident ended up saying that this guy looked like a major league
looney tune. Unfortunately, the patient overheard him. He went wild, criticizing the resident and asking to be transferred to another doctor. That's
when I got involved. He was still complaining of chest pain, so the nurses
were a little upset and didn't want to send him out thinking that he might

have heart disease. The guy was really pissed off that we were minimizing his complaints. It was 4 A.M. by this time, and I was only half conscious myself, and here he is showing me all these pieces of scotch tape with all these little things on them.

He had a pocket microscope, which he took out and made me look through, which I stupidly did... and I listened to all his complaints in great detail for almost two hours. We even did an EKG on him to play it safe. It was perfectly normal, so I sent him out. At that point, he was criticizing me even more than the first doctor. It was hard to get a word in edgewise to examine him because he had this stream of words pouring out, including all the famous doctors he knew and how much trouble he could get me into.

I handled this in a very stupid way. I just got trapped. I knew better at the time but just couldn't handle it. I should have booted him right out. I was trying to be patient and I got misused; I even ended up prescribing a medicine that's fairly harmless for scabies just to get rid of him.

The danger with situations like that is they can make you careless. I remember this man who came in with belly pain. I did the standard tests but decided against getting a flat plate [x-ray] of his abdomen because it didn't seem very serious. You see so much abdominal pain that you get desensitized to it. It just looked like one of those intestinal virus type of things. I sent him home with some mild medication to relieve spasm... and I found out a few days later he had been admitted to another hospital for emergency surgery because he had a small bowel obstruction. I kind of got raked over the coals by an attending surgeon in the ER because of this. In front of the group including the nurses, he put me through a quiz about small bowel obstruction, asking me questions like I was a third-year med student. It was humiliating. I won't miss the next one.

Eventually, I do shake these things off, but they bother me for a while. You don't like to make these kinds of mistakes. People can die. Now I get a flat plate on every abdominal patient... including a lot that probably aren't needed. You're sort of caught between missing a diagnosis and doing too many lab tests. If you order too many tests, the worst you get is a slap on the wrist. If you miss an important diagnosis, you really catch hell. It makes us all, supercautious, expensive kind of doctors.

We probably could use some emergency medicine residents in the ER, but we don't have any because it's controlled by the department of medicine. I don't really understand the issues. It's some kind of territorial battle. I think it's inappropriate for us to be running the ER, even though we learn a lot there. We have one of the best emergency medicine programs in the country... it's cited as a model. It's really beyond me. Anyway, I've got all I can cope with. I can't deal with any more problems right now.

I know there's a lot of talk about house officers having easy access to drugs and using them to handle the stress and fatigue. There may be a bit of it but I have never seen it directly. These people have been through too much and are much too smart to get involved in anything illegal. Alcohol is a different matter. There are lots of people drinking more than they should, and I know it's tension-related. But the house officers don't have any corner on that. I could name a few attendings who are into the sauce a good bit.

There isn't even a lot of temptation for me to drink. With most of my friends and my fiancée hundreds of miles from here, I don't have much social life to speak of. I read. I exercise. I talk to her on the phone. You don't have that much time anyway.

I spend a lot of time thinking about the future and what our life will be like. That's one of the important things that gets me through this. I know it's time-limited and there are a lot of better days coming.

▲   ▲   ▲

Although the house officers in this group experienced a good deal of satisfaction with much of the sophisticated teaching they receive and from the work with complex clinical problems, they also seemed to be chafing about some issues that they found troubling and unresolvable. They were, as are many young people, caught up in the dilemma of wanting more freedom and more responsibility while often being a bit frightened and wary of having to provide leadership for junior colleagues and irritated by attendings who didn't make sufficient investment in teaching. This ambivalence about one's own dependency appears repeatedly in house officer interviews throughout this book.

Also, they labored with complicated patients who made demands that seemed to be illogical and unanswerable and to have nothing to do with any organic disorder. They wanted to be presented with severe pathology that would lend itself to decision-free rational thinking and that wasn't muddied up by the patient's social problems and emotional needs. They were totally unaware that there was nothing in their training to help them understand how to interpret these apparently unrealistic demands and to deal with them more responsibly.

Dr. D. who was a 29 year old senior resident, seemed finally able to bring some perspective to the roller coaster of dependency and independency that he had experienced for so many years. He stated,

▼   ▼   ▼

In retrospect, it's funny how you progress. It's not a smooth curve. Like on June 24 of your internship year, you go off for a week's vacation. Up until then, you've been doing your work and taking orders. People tell you what to do. You have a little freedom, but not much. You come back from vacation, and there, standing in front of you, are three totally green interns and some third-year medical students waiting for your orders. All of a sudden, you're the boss. It's kind of a shock. It's a very interesting period in your life. Initially, you're scared, but you don't show it. It's so much better... finally... BOOM... you're in charge. You ask yourself how can they put me in this position? I'm not ready for this. But you really are and that's a good feeling. My life improved 300-fold in that week I went from intern to resident.

I think the way you get through an internship is you've already had a lot of experiences that are not as bad, but similar. You were a big-shot senior in high school and suddenly you were a college freshman, which is lower than nothing. Then you were a college senior and became a freshman in medical school and realized how ignorant you were. Finally, you got to be a senior in med school, and your family and friends thought you were God's gift to medicine. Then the house of cards comes crashing down: you're an intern in a big teaching hospital, and for a while, it seems like every nurse knows more than you do. So, you've had a lot of experience on this roller coaster of self-esteem, and you just ride with it. Your skin gets pretty thick in the process.

▲   ▲   ▲

The cold bath that comes at the beginning of most internships creates a sharp-edged awareness of this problem with suddenly acquired responsibilities (often in life-or-death situations) and past longings for freedom. Dr. A., in her first year of internal medicine training as an intern, described her complex feelings:

▼   ▼   ▼

I remember very clearly what it was like to go from student to intern. You wait for years for the time when you can write the orders on the patient and be listened to. It's not so bad during the day when there are lots of residents and attendings around, and you can always grab one if you're in trouble. It's the nights when you're more-or-less alone. There are people on call, but in emergencies you can't wait 10 or 15 minutes for someone to come.

One night, when I was on cardiology, I was standing in the hall about 2 A.M., and they grabbed me and said this guy had gone into ventricular fibrillation. So, here I am in this room with three nurses and a patient I never saw before in my life, who's now going into cardiac arrest. I didn't know anything about him... why he was in the hospital... not even his name. He wasn't even on our service. He was a cardiac surgery patient. But I shocked him... more than once... and he woke up and I said how do you do. I never did know much about him, but I did this horribly invasive procedure on him. You just respond and hope you know enough to be doing the right thing because sometimes you're it and you can't hide behind being a student anymore. Those days when you complained about how hard you were working seem like kid stuff now.

▲   ▲   ▲

The stream of patients who traditionally come into the emergency room at odd hours and who present unusual, puzzling, or irrational complaints left most of these house officers irritated and frustrated. Dr. S.'s anger at the third-year medical student who wanted help at 5 A.M. with a bad cold and with the emotionally disturbed patient who claimed he had scabies was a frequently expressed emotion. There was little or no help from more senior residents or from attendings, who also seemed to have scant knowledge about how to deal with these patients.

Dr. D.'s description of his experience reinforces this point.

▼   ▼   ▼

Outside of the real trauma cases, a lot of what you see is people with a heavy combination of physical and psychological problems. Who knows why they suddenly decide at 3 A.M. that the sore throat they've had for weeks is now much worse and needs immediate attention? Probably some psychological stressor triggers something in their heads and they have to come in at that point.

You get pissed off when this happens in the middle of the night and you are losing a lot of sleep, but you can't show it to the patient. You probably get rid of him more quickly. You move him in and out. Then you go to the back office and let off steam to the other house officers or the nurses. But you definitely don't show it to the patient. It's much worse when you're an intern because you get called so much more often. I'm amazed at how quickly I put this behind me and don't think about it much anymore . . . and how stressful it was then to be constantly exposed to that kind of behavior. You just think: Why would any normal person come into the ER with this kind of complaint at this time? You calmly ask the patient what the problem is, and then you go off to the nursing station and you say, 'Goddamn that stupid son-of-a-bitch. I can't believe this guy is here at three o'clock in the morning with a sore throat.'

Then, there's what you call the 'suitcase sign.' We had one yesterday morning. He came in at 7 A.M. with a history of constipation and rectal bleeding for 20 years. He was going on a fishing trip in a few days and didn't want to be bothered with it. He heard somewhere we had a specialist in this field. He had gotten up at four o'clock and had driven 150 miles so he could be the first in line to be admitted. There he stood, with his suitcase, wanting to come into the hospital to have his constipation fixed. I knew we were in for it when the nurse came back and told me we had a patient with a positive suitcase sign. He turned out to be a guy in his 60s who wasn't even really constipated, and we couldn't find any blood on the rectal exam. He was just one of those individuals who thought he ought to have at least one bowel movement a day, and if he didn't, then there was something wrong with him. He left the ER a very dissatisfied customer.

▲   ▲   ▲

Eventually, what the house officers described was that they had developed techniques for stonewalling or ditching patients without getting emotionally involved with them. This tendency to withdraw from involvement with emotionally disturbed people, distressed families, or dependent patients is an important defense and a necessary one in the absence of better clinical skills for dealing with this population.

Some house officers entertained the stereotype that poor or uneducated patients are harder to deal with because they don't comprehend or are not able to follow instructions. They planned to work in suburbia with middle-class or upper-class families, who they felt would be more compliant. Conversely, there was a smaller group of house officers who saw this more affluent group differently. For instance, Dr. A. said about her future plans, "As I think of the future, I see myself in a general medical practice in the inner city. I can't see myself in academic medicine or out in the high-rent district. Well-to-do people are too hard to take care of. They don't listen and they're not grateful. Poor people are easier to take care of. They listen to you, and you can tell them what's wrong and help them. I get along a lot better with those people. Maybe it goes back to my peasant stock. I don't like to coddle wealthy people. They are always reading and coming to you with lots of other opinions, and my son the doctor says this and my uncle the doctor wants to know why you don't do this test and that kind of crap. In the end, there are 30 opinions, and they don't listen to you or do what you tell them to anyway. That's not for me."

The characteristics of the patient population generally cared for by physicians in this specialty (in contrast to surgery, for instance) is that they usually present long-term, chronic problems, often with mixed diagnoses, often demonstrating slow progress in response to treatment. Nevertheless, the appeal for many of the house officers lay in this long-term responsibility. This was again in marked contrast to most of the surgical house officers, who enjoyed a practice in which rapid assessment, speedy intervention, and quick resolution of the clinical problem were the most appealing features.

Again, Dr. A., a medical intern only a few months from medical school, described the attraction of this work: "The other experience we have during this first year is our continuity clinic. That's why I was late for our appointment. I like it a lot. You can get to know the patients and follow them for a period of time. It's not exciting or dramatic stuff—you know, hypertension, diabetes, chronic kidney disease, and the like. For most of the people, it's really a matter of keeping them out of the hospital. You're doing a lot for them if you do that. You don't hit any home runs. There is no magic. Most of them have long-term chronic diseases, and you do very well if you can keep them at home and working, if possible. A lot of them are little old ladies that have six or seven things wrong with them. I'm a big fan of not putting them in the hospital. It's not the place for them. They pick up infection and go downhill, or they sit around and have their pulmonary emboli. I'll do anything to keep them out of the hospital."

Despite her tender years, Dr. A. captured in a few words what many practitioners of internal medicine find most compelling about the work despite their lack of knowledge of family dynamics in any formal sense and their feelings of inadequacy in the face of patients who make demands on their time and energy because they suffer from undiagnosed psychological problems.

Chapter 3

PEDIATRICS

Dr. Q. is a 26-year-old second-year resident in pediatrics. She joined me in my office at noon, having come across the street from the Children's Hospital, where she was now assigned to the emergency room. We talked at first through our BLTs, which I had ordered, wolfing them down in a few minutes and sipping away at the hot, acidic coffee that had been steeping in my outer office since 7:30 A.M. She was pleasant, cheerful, outgoing, and rarely at a loss for words. She seemed to enjoy the interview and to be pleased that anyone would really want to know the details of her daily life as a house officer. She was well groomed and dressed in whites that revealed only the rim of her crisp yellow shirt collar.

▼   ▼   ▼

The way the system works, this is my fourth stint in the emergency room. In your second year, you spend five rotations there. Each is three weeks long. You're sort of in charge when you're there, but you can always get help if you need it. On some of the assignments, you're in the ER from 10 P.M. until 7 A.M. On those shifts, you are pretty much on your own. But even then, there are subspecialty residents in the house like in cardiology or neurology, so you can always get another opinion if you get stuck. They pretty much cushion you there. Sometimes, you feel a little overprotected.

The time when you really feel sort of exposed is when you go out on transport; that's when there's an infant in very critical status at some outlying community hospital that doesn't have all the specialists and all the high-tech hardware you need to save these tiny babies—like a pound and a half. It's your job to go in the transport vehicle and make sure the baby gets back here still in viable condition. At first, I was absolutely terrified. I was overwhelmed by all these rescue fantasies that I couldn't fulfill. Eventually, one of the senior residents told me that no one expected that kind of thing. My job was just to keep the baby in stable condition until definitive care could be done. It's still tense work, but I'm more comfortable now because I know what's expected. I haven't had any catastrophes. I feel I can keep any condition stable if I have enough time and right equipment.

You change and grow so fast in all of this. If you don't, you can't survive. When I think back just to the beginning of this year, which was only eight months ago, I can remember my first day in the ER. As I said, if you're a second-year resident, you're in charge. It's almost funny now, but I didn't have the vaguest idea what that meant. I had worked in the same emergency room as an intern, but then you have almost no responsibility. Now, interns and nurses were turning to me for rapid decisions and for direction. I tried to hide just how frightened I was.

In retrospect, I think, I was more frightened by the staff than by the responsibility for knowing what was right in a medical sense. I didn't know how aggressive or how passive I should be. I remember one of the senior residents coming in and literally taking me by the hand and forcing me to take over. What an incredible transition has to take place in just a few days. You've spent your whole life being a student and suddenly somebody sticks a baton in your hand and tells you to lead the orchestra.

I'll never forget the first time I had to run a code red on a kid who had stopped breathing in the ICU. I really didn't feel like I knew what I was doing. Fortunately, there were people around who did. As you go along in the program, it gets to be the opposite: you feel there are too many people around, and you want more control.

These two sides of you are constantly battling with each other. If they bring an older child into the ER who is in severe respiratory distress and needs immediate intubation and you can't get the damn thing in place because he's struggling so, it's nice to call somebody down from anesthesia or the ICU who does it so smoothly. Or if they bring a kid in who is in such profound shock that all the surface veins are collapsed and you can't get an IV started, it's nice to be able to call a surgical resident because they know how to cut down on an artery and get a line in quickly.

There's this constant striving for autonomy while being secretly thankful that you've got all these experts around to bail you out when you're in trouble. I guess the ideal thing is to have them on call in the background without having them looking over your shoulder all the time. If they do, you really don't learn from your mistakes. Once, I sent a kid with sickle-cell anemia home from the ER with an outpatient appointment. When the attending reviewed the chart later, it was clear from the lab reports that he should have been admitted to the hospital right away. We got the patient in, and nobody really raised hell with me. They didn't have to. I punished myself enough—and I won't make that mistake again.

I've been talking as if this second year is all emergency room. Only about one fourth of it is. You get to spend time on other units, like the metabolic ward and other specialty services, and four months on the neonatal service at the obstetrical hospital. That includes working in the well-baby nursery, in the neonatal intensive care unit, and in the delivery room. For me, that was the most stressful part of the training so far. Especially at night, you're very much on your own. You can get an attending to come. They never say no, but it can take 10 or 15 minutes, and you usually don't have that much time in these life-and-death situations, especially with premies. And there you are in an operating room with a surgeon (the obstetrician) and an anesthesiologist—but they are absolutely no help. They will be the first to tell you that they're very good with adults but don't know much about two-pound premature infants.

I'll never forget the time I was having such trouble intubating this tiny preemie and the anesthesiologist tried to help. She threw up her hands. The patient was so tiny and the equipment was so difficult that she just felt inept. It was terrible. You feel so responsible for this little life. I was soaked with sweat. I kept trying until I got it. I realized there had been no heartbeat for six minutes, but somehow I got him out of it. That was a nightmare because most of the problems you see in preemies can be traced back to lack of oxygen. Of course, I only got to see him in the hospital. You don't know the long-range effects of this over the child's development.

I've noticed how little contact we have with families as residents around these catastrophes or near catastrophes. The attendings do it—but no one tells you how to handle it. There's no teaching around this. We even know who some of the high-risk ones are ahead of time. It would be nice if, when they first come into the hospital before delivery, we had a chance to meet them and talk and there is some rapport and some trust.

The worst day of my life, certainly since I've been an adult, happened in that OB hospital. There was this patient who, according to her obstetrician, was at 24 weeks' gestation, and there had been many serious complications during the pregnancy. Apparently, both her doctor and the nurses had told this mother that there was no way the baby could live. I found this out later. The mother delivered precipitously in her bed while being wheeled to the delivery room.

I was paged to come and pronounce the baby dead—which I also didn't realize. When I arrived a couple of minutes later, there they all were standing around the baby in the hallway. They had called me three minutes after the baby was born, and I could pick up a heartbeat. So I started to resuscitate the infant, using mouth to mouth since I had nothing else. I asked for help from the OB nurses, and they just walked away. The doctor leaned over and whispered that a decision had already been made not to try to resuscitate the baby.

There I stood. Nothing had been set up to resuscitate. No one would help. The mother was fully conscious, watching, listening, and wondering what was going on. The baby was gasping and had a very faint heartbeat. Morally, I felt this was a viable baby and that this was my decision, not the obstetrician's—who, by the way, was at least 20 years my senior and an associate professor. So I went for it. In the middle of all that confusion, I ran to the nearest phone, called the ICU for some neonatal nurses, and we finally got the baby back to the nursery.

The heart rate started to come up, and the other signs began to improve. The baby started to breathe by himself on a ventilator. I sat up with him all night. At 7 A.M. my attending pediatrician came by. I was extremely upset at this point because I had had a lot of time to think about what had happened and what my behavior had been. I was crying and I was angry. They should either have called me immediately when the baby had a better chance—or 15 minutes later to pronounce him dead. They got me into a Catch-22 where I couldn't do anything except try to save the baby, but by the time I really could intervene effectively, the baby had been oxygen-deprived so long it had to be badly damaged.

I tried to explain to my attending what had happened and how hard it had been to make the decision with no support. He went and talked to the mother and then the obstetrician. He decided to pull the plug. Several hours later, the baby died. It was never discussed with me. That part's okay. Maybe I would have done the same thing as an attending given the same circumstances. It turned out that the baby had a bad skull fracture and a lot of other complications. It would have been an extremely impaired infant if it had survived at all.

What had me off the wall was the way the entire thing went. We are trained from Day 1 that when you go into the delivery room and there are any signs of life in the baby, you just proceed to do what you know how to do in order to sustain life. Later on, when there's time, you can consider together with the parents what the future risks are and what should be done from that point. There should have been a neonatal consultation on this case when the mother first came into the hospital. We should have been filled in, and we should have been prepared for what happened. I shouldn't have been called to run into that situation blind.

Here's a mother who's already given up her baby, and she sees this agitated young doctor trying to raise the infant from the dead. We talked later, and she said that she hoped everything that could have been done for the baby was done. Well...it wasn't. I carried that guilt around for days. [Her eyes filled up.] God, I still can't talk about it without getting very emotional.

My pattern of handling this kind of thing when I get very upset is to talk, talk, talk—with my fellow residents, with family, with friends. I guess it's a kind of confessional. It helps to relieve my guilt. Then, I try to walk away from it and tell myself I've learned and will do better next time.

My buddies told me it wasn't my fault, that I had done everything I could. That's not true. If that ever happens again, you can bet your sweet bippy that I won't be standing around in the hallway debating matters with a bunch of people who don't know much about it and don't have the responsibility anyway. I wasn't deliberate enough, not aggressive enough. I will snatch that kid up and run to the nearest ICU, and in 30 seconds, we'll have him on the right life-support system. Then and only then will we talk about it. And it will happen again. Other residents have told me about many similar situations where they have been caught like this.

I hope the obstetrician learned something, too. If you're convinced that you have a nonviable baby, you should not implicate the pediatrician. Call him 10 or 15 minutes later when it's all over.

Just recounting that incident probably tells you something about how I chose pediatrics as a specialty. It's maybe more a matter of temperament than anything else. As you go through med school, you find yourself identifying with different personality types that seem to go into different specialties. I'm more like the pediatricians. I'm not an adult doctor, and I'm certainly not the surgical type. That leaves pediatrics. We have a lot of the kid still in us. We're not so heavy. We're more relaxed and laid back. We enjoy playing and laughing. And the practice is mostly young, healthy little kids who are fun to be with. It's true that we see some very serious problems, but they are the exceptions. The average pediatrician with a big practice rarely has more than a couple of kids in the hospital at any one time.

As I think about the future, I'm torn between that kind of practice and taking a fellowship in developmental pediatrics and going the full-time academic route. I'm curious about what really happens to all these two-pound babies that we 'save.' Do they really make it later? How do they function? Are we doing them any favors by saving them? Or are we just creating untold misery for them and their families? None of the studies seem to follow these kids beyond a year or two. That's not enough. What is their life like in school and with friends? I would like to take a good close look at that.

You wanted to know what I have found the most stressful about this training. Well, I think the incident I described earlier is a good example of the kind of acute stress you encounter. In some ways, the chronic stresses are worse. First of all, it's hard to do anything about them. One of them is the chronic fatigue and sleep deprivation. These make you irritable, and then it's harder to make good decisions, to feel sure of yourself and to have any kind of life outside the hospital. If you have weaknesses, they tend to be magnified when you're exhausted.

I guess the other thing is the frequent anger over feeling totally out of control of things. The hospital is being reorganized now and we have no input. It's very stressful. There's no one to listen to you. The chief resident sort of works for the medical director. He doesn't represent us. We could suggest things that could make life a lot easier for everyone, but the system doesn't listen to house officers. When a bunch of sick kids control your life and your schedule, sometimes you get angry because you've lost one kind of control. But when a mindless bureaucracy just doesn't listen, then you're furious.

It would help if you could have some life outside of here, but it's hard to separate your personal and professional lives. They're constantly affecting each other. It's tough to be a single female resident and date people. Your exposure is to the people you work with all day. It's hard to meet anyone outside. And if you do, your schedule is so limited. When you do find something you want to do and someone you want to do it with and the time to do it, you never know whether you'll be able to get out of the hospital in time—or, even if you do, whether you'll be so darn tired that you won't be wide awake enough to enjoy it.

▲   ▲   ▲

Accepting responsibility for the life and well-being of a vulnerable infant or child, even partial responsibility, is awesome. The format of training in pediatrics seems to be set up in such a way as to provide a hierarchy of supervision so that, during the more junior years, constant oversight and consultation are available. In fact, house officers in other specialties, like neurosurgery, neurology, and family practice, tended to complain that they were treated as junior interns when they are on their rotation in pediatrics (as it applied to their particular specialty). They perceived an atmosphere in which the children were almost "protected" from mismanagement or exploitation by heartless physicians who didn't appreciate the sensitivities of childhood.

Nevertheless, the transition from year to year in pediatric training may still be experienced as frightening to house officers because it carries with it more and more responsibility, not only for children and their families, but for more junior trainees. Although this is generally true in all specialties, it seems to be more acutely felt in pediatrics. Whether this is in the nature of the training or of the trainees themselves cannot be discerned from the interviews available in this book.

Predictably, all pediatric house officers agreed that their greatest stress was in dealing with a dying child and with the parents. One might guess that this would become a bit easier with more experience and greater clinical skills in counseling the child and the parents. This appears not to be the case. Dr. McD., a 29-year-old senior resident, explained it to me this way:

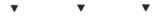

I've observed kind of a funny phenomenon, both in myself and in others. Most of us go into pediatrics because we like kids and we enjoy working with them. So you sort of expect, early on, that you're going to be badly clobbered when little kids die on you. Strangely enough, this seems to be more of a problem as time goes along than it is at the beginning. Like, during the first few months of your internship, you're so overwhelmed by the sheer volume of work and the complexity of the services that you can't react to kids as people.

By the end of the year, you are more on top of things and you start seeing the patients as real kids and the reality of it all starts to come down on you, especially if the kid dies or is permanently disabled. At the beginning, you don't realize the social implications. It's just, 'Oh, here's another leukemia.' Also, toward the end of the year, you are so fatigued and spaced out that you are more irritable and your threshold to stress is lower. A lot of your initial verve and idealism is stripped away because you know what is coming with a lot of these kids. You've been through it several times and you know there is no magic.

Part of the stress is that you work so hard with these kids trying to save them and they go through so much and then you end up with the result that you could have had in the first place without all your work and all their agony. You really wonder about it. When death finally happens, it's almost a relief. Sometimes, it's the ones who survive that are even worse tragedies because you know what kind of life they and their families have ahead of them.

One of the particularly tough parts of it is that most kids don't die acutely, like adults do from coronaries and strokes. They die slow deaths, like with leukemia or cystic fibrosis. They have impressions of what their death will be like, and they ask you questions if they are older. I try to be somewhat obtuse in my answers because you really don't know when it's going to happen or how it's going to happen. I think it's better to answer in generalities.

▲   ▲   ▲

Dr. McD. put his finger very nicely on an important dynamic. The capacity to deny both external and internal realities when faced with new experiences and with demands to master novel skills is a phenomenon with which we are all familiar. It is not uncommon to look back on a very trying period and to wonder how we got through it earlier in life, when, in fact, the capacities for denial made it possible to filter out threatening or disorganizing knowledge and to concentrate on the immediate tasks at hand. Only later did we permit reality to impinge on us.

Dr. I., a 25-year-old married pediatric intern, found herself pregnant during the last part of her senior year in medical school and the first half of her internship. Faced almost daily with caring for physically damaged and developmentally disabled children, she was able to maintain an optimistic attitude about her pregnancy. She said, "The other thing that deɲial helped me do was completely separate the idea that I was carrying this little baby in my belly from those terribly damaged infants that I was taking care of every day. There was never a thought like 'Oh God, this could happen to me!' In general, I just didn't act like a pregnant lady in front of my colleagues and the nurses. My pride wouldn't let me put them in the position where they might be expected to treat me as special or more needy. I'm a very private person."

Most residents seem able to do this. Failing to do it, especially so early in training, might well result in decompensation accompanied by depression and even paralysis of action.

Toward the end of training, residents are able to settle for partial goals, to relate to the positive aspects of the child and the family, and to give up their magical rescue fantasies. This reaction permits them to look at the child more as a real person and to experience less of an all-or-none reaction to the child's catastrophic illness and impending death. Dr. McD. described his current relationship with a young cancer patient as follows:

▼   ▼   ▼

What I'm finding most rewarding is when you take care of a difficult kid for a long period of time and it works out well. I have this teenager who comes frequently for chemotherapy, and we have gotten to know each other. We have lots of common interests, like sports. This is a long-term thing and he is my patient. I think I have given him the very best care he could get anywhere, and I've made a very positive impact on his life. I see a lot of him and I know everything about him, even little things like what is going on in school, problems with his skin, and changes in the flexibility of his limbs. We just deal with every little thing as it comes up.

For me, this is the good part of pediatrics. I've always liked working with kids. I don't mind the screaming and the yelling and having a difficult time with a kid. I also like the preventive aspect of pediatrics, which is not so true in the adult field. Most kids actually get better. I couldn't be more pleased with my choice of specialty. I'm happier every day with it.

▲   ▲   ▲

Until the day arrives when the resident can function in this way, one sees a tendency to relate to the disease as the object of concern, rather than the child because attachment to and subsequent loss of the child are unbearable.

One resident described his experience of working in the neonatal intensive care with severely damaged neonates as follows:

▼   ▼   ▼

I dealt with the stress of working in the neonatal ICU in kind of a funny way. There, you have these tiny babies dying on you frequently. In my head, these just didn't seem like kids to me. This probably sounds terrible, but they look like little primates, not human beings, and somehow you don't relate to them like you do to a kid. My feeling is, if we weren't there and the unit wasn't there, these kids would die, so we are doing something that 15 or 20 years ago was impossible and that makes me feel good.

In the end, most of them do okay, although I know there are some that turn out to be real train wrecks. So I didn't find it hard. They kind of look like little animals in this place. Sometimes, I think if we were suddenly covered by a volcanic eruption and they dug out the neonatal ICU five thousand years later, they would see all these little creatures in these glass bubbles. They would wonder if it was some sort of tomb...or a place of worship. You know, we worship these little creatures in these glass bubbles.

▲   ▲   ▲

This ability to depersonalize the child, although in some ways it may compromise the quality of interpersonal care, makes it possible for the house officer to survive psychologically when there are few other supports in his or her life.

Although technical support may be high, psychological support and guidance are experienced as low by pediatric house officers in general. Dr. C., a 24-year-old pediatric intern, said,

▼   ▼   ▼

My contract was renewed for next year, which I guess is a kind of positive feedback, but there is nothing specific. We don't know where to concentrate. When I don't know enough about my shortcomings, then I get shaky. I know the attendings fill out evaluation sheets on us, but I never see them. For all I know, they end up in the wastebasket.

There's really no one in authority you can talk to. We see the chairman about once a week at morning report and at some social functions, and he's really very nice, but the department is so big and there are so many house officers that there is no chance for one-to-one contact. Besides, this is the man who is going to be writing letters of recommendation for you later on, and you can't let him see too many of your deficiencies or start looking like a bellyacher. I've been to the chief resident about some of my problems, but I didn't get very far. His priority is to make sure everything gets done. He just changed the subject and deflected what I was saying. I can't say that he is terribly interested in the house officers' welfare. What this program should have is a chief resident who puts a higher priority on helping house officers who are starting out or a junior faculty member to do this.

I think some of the people are using too much alcohol to handle the stress, and I'm probably one of them. I use a little pot, too. There ought to be better ways. I'm not proud of it, but there is no time or energy for the kinds of things I used to do, like exercising or jogging or reading for pleasure.

▲   ▲   ▲

The stress of trying to deal with distraught and sometimes inappropriately angry parents is a chronic one, and one for which there is comparatively little preparation in training. Dr. Q., whose interview opened this chapter, was particularly concerned about this. Dr. McD., from whom we have heard previously, added, "No one teaches you how to handle this stuff either with parents or inside your own head. I guess you sort of learn it in the college of hard knocks. It's especially tough in the ER, where you're working pretty much alone. On the inpatient units, the attendings and the social workers handle a lot of this stuff with the parents. But when it comes time for you to handle it, you're on your own."

One house officer agreed that he had been fairly critical of parents who gave him a hard time until his own child became sick. He went on to say,

▼   ▼   ▼

My wife and I were absolutely frantic. I was a total wreck. We bothered people a lot and probably made pains out of ourselves. I never fully appreciated this before. Now, I react to parents differently as a result of that experience. You feel totally out of control. My daughter was only about 15 months old then and couldn't really communicate. You're in the next room and you hear your kid screaming and you wonder what's going on. It was bad enough for me as a pediatrician. Imagine what other parents must be thinking as they listen.

Now I understand what parents mean when they say they feel frustrated with the whole thing and they just want to leave and walk out. You kind of feel like there is nothing you can do. These other people have control and you're helpless. Often parents in the ER say, 'I want to leave here. I don't want to have anything to do with you people anymore.' They get very frustrated. They just feel they are not the parents anymore and are not in control of their children's lives. The best thing you can do is give them something to do so they can feel useful. I even felt better when they let me back in the examining room and I could pick up my kid and give some comfort and act like a father.

If there's one patient I had to pick out as sticking in my head, it's this little 10-year-old girl I had to take care of when I was an intern over two years ago. She had leukemia. She was really at the end of her course. There was nothing more we had to offer her except pain relief from all the hemorrhaging into her bones. We had an IV morphine drip going 24 hours a day. The day before she died, she started to have visions of her casket and her hearse. It was very bizarre and very upsetting.

You would go by her room, and she would be sitting up and she would say, 'I see my casket. I see it. It's right here.' I couldn't avoid her room because she needed so much attention. Her parents had a very difficult time. They couldn't face it and sort of pulled out completely. They'd had a tough time dealing with the disease from the beginning, and when this happened, they just bailed out, and I was stuck with it, along with the nurses. Finally, we turned up her morphine drip and put her into a semicoma, and the visions stopped. I guess we did it more for us than for her.

▲   ▲   ▲

Locus-of-control issues sometimes become paramount for a house officer, especially in pediatrics. One is dealing largely with a population of children, with whom it is very difficult to reason if they are very young. Parents can become, as we have seen, either extremely demanding or emotionally detached if the stress becomes unbearable. The need of the physician to be in control of the situation—to be able to call the shots and to have some sense that he or she is determining the outcome—is almost inbred. When the system in which the house officer is working and learning is perceived as unresponsive or out of control, frustration can mount, as Dr. Q. described in her interview.

Yet, thousands of young people are attracted to this field each year. Why? Despite the frustrations, the system issues, and the nagging sense that one does not know enough to deal with many of these children, for most, the rewards more than compensate, as Dr. Q. told us: "We have a lot of the kid still in us. We're not so heavy. We're more relaxed and laid back. We enjoy playing and laughing. And the practice is mostly young, healthy little kids who are fun to be with." All of the pediatric house officers I interviewed agreed with that statement.

BIBLIOGRAPHY

There is almost no need to look further than the following reference. This conference, attended by many of the leaders in pediatric training, summarizes the findings of most studies up to that time, and in a series of carefully edited presentations and discussions, the reader will find detailed information about the current state of our knowledge in this particular area, together with some of the approaches now being used to prevent burnout in pediatric house officers. Highly recommended.

Hoekelman, RA (Chairman): Stress in Pediatric House Staff Training, Proceedings of a Conference Sponsored by the Study Group on Pediatric Education and Ross Laboratories, March 5–7, 1985, Point Clear, AL.

Chapter 4

PSYCHIATRY

Dr. J. is a 27-year-old second-year resident in psychiatry. He appeared at ease. He was dressed in a loud checked shirt and a very narrow bright green tie. Through much of our meeting he kept an unlit, thin cigar with a plastic mouthpiece between his teeth.

▼   ▼   ▼

Right now, I'm working on an inpatient unit for kids and adolescents with autism or severe developmental problems. This is about my fifth or sixth rotation. I've been on the mood disorders unit, the acute adolescent service, neurology, the diagnostic center, and the schizophrenia inpatient service.

You're talking to me at a good time if you want to know something about survival skills in this training program. The last two days have been very hectic. Today is a good example. It starts at 7:30 with morning report from the night nurses, then ward rounds, and then I have to meet with my attending to go over any major problems and discuss new admissions. All these cases are tough and confusing. This morning, we must have spent over half the time talking about this one 11-year-old girl who really scares the hell out of me. She's nonverbal and spends most of her time, if you let her, banging her head on the wall or rocking and humming. She requires one-on-one nursing care, and even then, she has managed to hurt herself a few times. To try to protect her head, we've got her in a football helmet now. It's really kind of amusing to see this frail looking 11-year-old girl in this big helmet. But if you turn your back on her for 15 seconds, she manages to get out of it. She's so damn fast. I don't know how she does it. The trick will be to find the right combination of meds and behavior modification program that will eliminate these symptoms.

It's been hard for me to accept the fact that this is one disease [infantile autism] that we can't cure. At the moment, we're trying to prevent her from doing more damage to herself. Every time I think about how frustrated I feel, I think of the special-ed teachers, the nurses, and the other staff who spend so much more time with her than I do. What a tough way to make a living.

Oh, I had started to tell you about today. Well, by the time I finish checking in with my attending, it's about 9 A.M. and I know if I don't start writing progress notes, I'll catch hell. So, I spend most of the next hour at that. There has to be a detailed note on every patient every day.

Then the rest of the morning is spent seeing patients who need more attention than you can give them on rounds, reviewing treatment plans with ward staff, talking with families either in person or on the phone, updating medication orders—that kind of stuff.

Usually I can catch a quick lunch, but not today. The only time my family therapy supervisor can see me this week is going to take care of that. I'll pay for that later because I can get along without sleep if I have to, but not without food.

Then, the entire afternoon I have scheduled with outpatients, which is going to be fun because I just learned I will have a new admission on the unit about two o'clock. That's going to take an hour right out of the middle of the afternoon.

People really think you can be in two places at once, so they get a little pissed at you when you hold up the schedule. I'm learning to be fast on my feet. You can't keep everybody happy. When you're a medical student, even an intern, other people decide priorities for you. There's nobody to do that now. But it's my ass if I ignore the system too much.

Am I starting to sound a little disorganized? If I am, maybe that's because that's the way it is; most days are pretty chaotic and unpredictable.

If you were to ask me what is the hardest part of this training, that's it. You're dealing with the unpredictable human element all day. My friends who went into surgery or medicine think this is a low-pressure specialty. The drain on your mental energy is enormous. You're dealing with very disturbed, sometimes irrational patients, with very upset families—and with staff who are only human and have their breaking point, too. All of this has to be factored into your decisions about treatment.

And of course, as you move from service to service, you have to keep on shifting gears. It takes a different set of skills to be an effective psychiatrist on a unit for depressed suicidal adults than it does on one for primitive, regressed autistic kids. You can burn out. I have to keep telling myself, 'You've adapted to new situations before; you'll do it again. Give it time. Hang in there.' So far, I've been able to make the changes in how I think and function by remembering how I got this far.

[At this point in the interview, Dr. J.'s pager beeped insistently. There was a message from the head nurse to come to the unit stat. One of his patients was having a grand mal seizure. As he left, we agreed to meet again later the same day to complete our talk. What follows is the result of that contact. It was now the middle of the evening. He looked spent and was tieless and cigarless.]

Sorry I had to dash out like that today. We're having a hell of a time controlling this patient's seizures. Part of the problem with this teenager is that he is so oppositional that he gets very cute with his medication. He's become expert at cheeking it and then spitting it in the toilet. When you can fool the nurses on that floor, you're good.

I was trying to tell you about a typical day, and I don't think I got even halfway through it! I'm very tired now, but I actually feel pretty good. In spite of a lot of things that could have thrown me a year ago, I kept a level head today. When you make decisions and you see them working, you feel better and better—more confident.

Actually, I'm kind of a slow starter. I get up extremely early in the morning, have a quiet breakfast, and read the paper front to back before I come in. That settles me so I'm ready for the onslaught when it comes. I don't know if that's important, but you wanted to know about how I'm coping and that's part of my pattern.

Where did I leave off when I was trying to cover my day with you before? I guess I got up to about early afternoon when clinic started. I'm amazed now at what a distorted picture I had about what this specialty was like. I fantasized myself sitting in this comfortable easy chair while neurotic, articulate adults discussed their problems and hang-ups, and then we would figure ways to deal with these (with me having most of the answers, of course). Instead, what do I see this afternoon? A 19-year-old firesetter who burned down a suburban Woolworth's and is on five years' probation with psychiatric treatment as one of the conditions; a 38-year-old pregnant woman whose husband has left her and who is having very self-destructive thoughts and I'm trying to decide whether she's committable or not without saying anything to her about it; a 20-year-old kid who is mentally retarded and has these destructive temper outbursts where he trashes his room or wherever he is, and the agency who is responsible for him, his family, and the sheltered workshop where he spends most of the day are all in conflict over what to do about him; a 16-year-old anorexia nervosa who's down to 91 pounds and who is still complaining because she's too fat, and her obese mother sits in my office literally screaming because I won't make her eat. Should I go on?

Don't misunderstand me. This is terrifically exciting. It pushes my head up to the very limit. But it sure isn't as easy as it looks when you see it on TV.

Remember, in the middle of all this, I'm called back up to the ward to handle a new admission. On this service, there's a rule that all admissions must be seen by a physician within an hour of entry onto the unit, so I couldn't put it off. By 'handle,' I mean you have to review any preadmission studies or history that accompany the patient to the floor, you have to do a brief physical and mental status exam, you have to put an admission note on the chart, and you have to write orders. If you're fast and there are no interruptions, you can do it in an hour—while your patients sit in the clinic getting steamed because they think you're off somewhere drinking coffee or God knows what.

The new admission was something else again. I guess you have to be in this business 30 years before you begin to feel like you've seen it all. She turned out to be a young adult residual-type autistic—you know, infantile autism 25 years later. She was a transfer from surgery, where she had just had to have her anal sphincter and rectum repaired because she had inserted a ginger-ale bottle up there. The mental status exam was fascinating. She just kept on saying, 'Ginger-ale, ginger-ale, ginger-ale.'

When I finished with my last clinic patient, I had to go back and examine her more thoroughly and develop an initial treatment plan for the first 72 hours of hospitalization. The nursing staff is going to have a hell of a time with her because of the rectal surgery. It'll be messy, to put it mildly. Anyway, another hour and a half went into that.

Usually, I can get out of here by 7:00 or 7:30 P.M. Most week nights, I'm too pooped to do anything that takes a lot of thinking. I make myself some dinner and stare at the boob tube for an hour or two. Or I see some friends or talk on the phone with family. I know I haven't been pulling on retractors all day like the surgery residents have been, but I feel like I have. If you asked me what I saw on TV last night, I wouldn't be able to tell you. Professional reading has to be done early in the morning or not at all. I'm lucky if I can do one third of what I should. Thursday afternoons have been set aside as didactic seminar time. Various faculty members who specialize in certain areas lead discussions around certain clinical topics or the newest research. You should go to all of these. It's your last chance to be spoon-fed this way, but again, I can only get to about one out of three. You just pick and choose and go to the ones that are most interesting to you.

I know that when it comes time to take my board exams and I have to dig out all this stuff on my own, I'll be sorry, but if I went to every seminar, grand rounds, VIP lecture, or research conference that this place puts on, I'd be fired at the end of the year because my patients weren't getting the proper attention and my charts were not up-to-date. The truth of the matter is that I'd rather work with patients than sit in a conference room any day. Do you realize that I'm 28 and I have been going to school for 25 years! I'll be 30 before I earn my first dollar, and then I can start paying off my education loans.

Sorry, I sound like I'm bitching now, and I really shouldn't. Basically, I'm very happy with my choice both of medicine and psychiatry. I told you earlier that you had caught me at a tough time. What you're hearing is the result of almost no personal time, too many canceled dates, and no time for reading.

Even from the very first day of med school, I've never had any serious doubts. I think a big part of my intense interest in medicine came from the fact that, for about the first 15 years of my life, I had severe asthma. The constant contact with doctors—just watching what they did, what a difference they made to me, what my parents thought of them—got me so involved that I wanted to be like them.

There's a little tag end on this story that I haven't told you, though. It was obvious that, between asthmatic attacks, I really had some athletic ability. Without hardly trying, I could play the infield smoothly and instinctively know what to do with the ball when it was hit to me without being told. As a kid, I could hit the ball a couple of hundred feet. But always, the asthma came along, and there was never any chance to develop the talent or become a permanent part of a team.

Now the asthma is gone, but I'm 27 and that's all nothing but a fantasy. When I watch a big-league game on the tube, there's a sadness for me. I feel I belong out there with the rest of those guys. So it's a paradox. My chronic illness kept me out of one profession and got me into another. I'm determined to salvage some of that identity. This spring, I'm going to sign up for some body-building classes, and I'm even considering getting involved in a program like the martial arts. You're keeping a straight face, but I know you're probably smiling inside. Here's this kid psychiatrist who wants to become a karate expert. Laugh if you want to, but I'm determined not to give up the part of myself that got buried because I had to lie in bed breathing with a nebulizer, taking hundreds of allergy shots, and feeling very much left out of things.

The choice of psychiatry was another thing, however. I don't think you actually know why you make a choice like that—at least not this early in your career. I just know that all the other specialties seemed dull and boring. There's something too routine about them. Psychiatry is much more exciting. I know the old story about every patient is different, but I watched internists and pediatricians and surgeons during my third-year clinical clerkships. They were all too rushed and too busy with gall bladders and kidneys and hearts to ever find out anything about their patients that made one different from the others. As I watch some of the faculty members in this department, that's a lot closer to what I want to be 10 years from now.

You may be wondering what I mean by 'some of the faculty members.' It's just that some turn me on and some don't. During the time I've been here, I've probably been exposed to maybe 15 or 20 attendings. I go for the ones that make me think out treatment decisions and keep me on target. I have a tendency to fly too much by the seat of my pants. The one who brings me up short and forces me to explain my clinical decision and helps me when my hand has been called and I can't is who I go for. You also encounter attendings who you feel are working primarily for their own advancement and are not very invested in patient welfare. They're not fooling the residents. They only think they are.

Maybe it was during my second month here that I got into a thing with one of the faculty. I guess, basically, I was wrong because I was spending too much time with one patient at the expense of the others, and I got a dressing down by the ward chief in front of the head nurse. He shouldn't have done it that way. I was demolished for days and began to wonder if I was in the right field after all. I got so anxious, I couldn't sleep, and I think that's the closest I've come to getting into psychotherapy myself. But it's funny what happens at times like that for me. I just hung in there and worked my butt off. I toughed it out. I kept thinking of all the stress I've handled in the past. Gradually, things got better. I've learned I can cope.

▲   ▲   ▲

Writing about interviews with house officers in one's own specialty is an exercise in caution. I know, from having supervised scores of them over decades, that they come into the field in many ways less prepared for clinical practice than in almost any other specialty.

The linear, nonassociative thinking process that is taught in most courses in medical school is not the best clinical decision-making model in the face of deviant human behavior.

In addition, the kind of medical authority that is modeled by teachers and attendings in medical school often does not work very well with patients who have mixed feelings about authority and dependency.

Although psychiatry has moved more toward a biomedical mode of diagnosis and treatment during the last 10 or 15 years, many of the most fundamental precepts of practice still apply. The primary role of the physician with a psychiatric patient is the same as in other specialties, but the way in which this function is negotiated and contracted for may be quite different. Patients who are severely disturbed and whose judgment is impaired may not be able either to understand or to appreciate the significance of their disorder. They may be highly suspicious of the physician and of the family who contracted for her or his services. In some instances, their basic mode of problem resolution may be through resorting to violence, passive aggressiveness, or flight.

Therefore, the young psychiatric resident is confronted not only with having to master a new body of knowledge and skills, but with the more vexing problem of learning how to use these effectively with a group of patients who may not understand what needs to be done, whose resistance to intervention may be high or unpredictable, and whose compliance with routine procedures may vacillate between slavish submission and hostile defiance.

And then there is the problem of the deviance itself. Most medical students have grown up in fairly conservative, middle-class families in which conformity to societal norms is expected. They would not have been able to get through premedical and medical training otherwise. Now, they find themselves confronted with bizarre behaviors (like Dr. J.'s patient with the ginger-ale bottle) and are expected not only to accept this behavior nonjudgmentally but to help change it.

Yet, all residents will tell you that the major source of learning is the patient himself or herself. They become so immersed in the histories and current lives of their patients that there is no question that the patient does become the primary teacher and the attending becomes the guide who helps to place all of this information in context.

Dr. K. is an unmarried 25-year-old woman who was finishing up her first year in psychiatry as an intern. She was 11 months out of medical school and faced the following situation:

▼   ▼   ▼

The patient who is giving me the hardest time right now is someone I've been seeing as an outpatient until three days ago, when we had to sign him in as an emergency, involuntary patient.

I really thought I was riding high on this case, and it blew up in my face. I came very close to having to cancel this appointment with you because I have just spent two hours with his wife trying to put her back together after what happened earlier today. Three days ago, when he woke up he told his wife he was Jesus and that he hated all Jews. He told her she was a Jew (neither of them is), and he spit in her face. He told her he was sorry that Hitler had not killed all the Jews. His wife called me in tears from a neighbor's house. She was terrified because he was so irrational and has been violent in the past. We had the police pick him up on an emergency 72-hour commitment against his will. The other reason we decided to do this is that they have a four-year-old kid.

As you can imagine, he's very angry at both me and his wife. What took so long today was the amount of time I had to spend with the wife and the hospital's lawyer discussing options with her. He refuses to stay in the hospital voluntarily. We are going to have to release him today because the hearing officer decided he couldn't be detained involuntarily. He said that spitting in someone's face isn't violent behavior. Even though he has a history of violence, the fact that he hasn't done anything in the last few months makes it legally impossible to detain him.

That's the law. The hearing officer is just doing his job, I guess. You know you have to have a hearing before a hearing officer appointed by the mental health administrator within 72 hours to determine legal grounds for detainment, and the need for treatment doesn't seem to mean anything. The only thing they look for are acts or threats endangering self or others within the last week or 10 days. These hearing officers are lawyers with no clinical background. Their concern is with due process and the civil rights of the patient. I'm all for that—but my God, the people we are putting out on the streets because of this is a crying shame. So many of them need treatment badly, but because their judgment is poor and they are so lacking in insight, they are getting no treatment. It's terrible for their families, especially the kids.

I have to admit, this is the first time I've been really scared. I don't think he would actually do anything to me. I think there is some trust there. I've been working with him for several months. [Long pause.] If I were the hearing officer, I would have committed him. Maybe the system is more crazy than the patient.

This is a different kind of stress from the stuff I was talking about earlier. There is probably some very real physical danger. But you just live with it. It comes with the territory. I've been doing a lot of deep-breathing exercises and taking my pulse a lot during the last 24 hours. I was able to get eight hours' sleep last night, but it wasn't restful sleep. Even though this patient is very sick, he could hold himself together long enough to buy a gun. I'm not saying that he comes off as the Duke of Pittsburgh, but he can fool you.

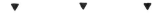

Then, later on in the same interview as she talked about her pediatric internship, which she had served in a large hospital adjacent to an inner-city ghetto elsewhere, she added, "I was more scared during parts of my internship than I am now. Many of the parents I saw in the emergency room were strung out on drugs and abusing their kids. They seemed a lot more dangerous to me than anyone I'm seeing now. And I'm more sure of myself now. I feel I understand better how to respond to an aggressive patient."

When you are 25 years old, bright and flexible, the coping mechanisms come into play rather quickly. This transition from "traditional" medical practice to psychiatry is more difficult for older residents who come into training having had several years of experience in another field. Although they usually come for sound reasons, they are also much more accustomed to the unquestioned authoritative role of the physician and the rather straight-line relationships between diagnosis and treatment in their former specialty.

Dr. Y., a 36-year-old second-year resident who had previously spent 10 years in the practice of internal medicine in a small town, described himself as a "retread." In discussing his transition to psychiatry, he said,

The difference between this professional life and the practice of internal medicine is beyond my powers of description. Before, I always felt I was operating from a position of authority. I don't mean like a policeman; I mean like an expert. Unfortunately, I was bored. I began to feel like a mechanic, like the technician who comes to fix your TV. I'm sure as hell not bored anymore. Not that there isn't some routine attached to this work. If you're a house officer in a big teaching hospital, there's always morning report, updating medication orders, and writing detailed progress notes on every patient every day. Those things take hours out of your schedule. It seems to me that one of the biggest problems in this field is the patient to whom you explain all the details and the reasons for pursuing a given course of treatment, and he sits there nodding his head, and then, there is no follow-through. Whether it's an absence of motivation or paralyzing ambivalence that prevents him from moving off the dime, I don't know. Sometimes, the family is so disorganized that they don't support the plan. It isn't acceptable to me to say, 'Well, you made a good try. If the patient won't use your help, that's his business.

You incur a responsibility when you take on a patient. It's ethical and legal. I've got a patient like that right now. He's depressed but not committable. We've talked a dozen times about the importance of taking his antidepressant medication and how much better he feels when he does. But he rarely takes it and he has lots of self-destructive thoughts. He's not in this alone. As his doctor, what kind of liability have I got if he does himself in because his treatment program isn't working? I find this very stressful. This is very different from what I was used to in the practice of medicine. This kind of thing isn't real to you until you confront it personally. Maybe the biggest surprise of all for me is the severity of sickness in these patients. It's so much more serious than I ever imagined.

We have one 19-year-old girl on the unit now who I think has been close to death a few times. She seems perfectly capable of starving herself to death if we don't intervene. I saw such cases when I was an internist, but I always referred them to a psychiatrist. Now, that's ME. Thank God I've got a faculty supervisor because this girl scares me. It's so irrational. I watch her stand in front of the mirror looking like something out of a concentration camp, and she whispers to herself that she looks like a cow and has to take off more weight!

▲   ▲   ▲

The psychiatry house officers, perhaps more than any other group, tended to make a clear distinction between what they saw as formal teaching and clinical supervision, on the one hand, and faculty support and guidance, on the other. These house officers seemed generally pleased with the kind of teaching and supervision they were receiving. They viewed their mentors as savvy, experienced, and articulate.

But surprisingly, considering the nature of the specialty itself, most viewed the faculty as rather oblivious to the stresses and pressures of training, and like the cobbler's children, they viewed themselves as walking around with holes in their emotional shoes.

Dr. G., a second-year resident who was in transition in this process, is a good person to close this discussion for us:

▼   ▼   ▼

Take this case I'm working with now. She's a 49-year-old woman who is depressed. I've been working with her for almost two years. She seemed like an ideal case to work with. She was intelligent, articulate, and well motivated. Not only that, she presented the possibility of learning to do psychotherapy, medication treatment, and family therapy all at once. There were a lot of areas in her life that were painful to her and that she wanted to change. Slowly, I've come to realize that she was the person who had developed this lifestyle and that she had done it for a reason. There were a lot of things she couldn't give up even though they were painful. I have fought harder against this realization, I think, than she has.

It's not as simple as just accepting the patient's limited goals for change; it's accepting those goals when you know so much more is possible. This woman has tremendous strengths, but most of them are bound up in conflicts with family members who don't want what she's got to offer, and she continues to struggle with them to get some kind of recognition or feedback that she's an important person in their lives.

I know I'm still doing a good job with her, but I'm not looking for basic change anymore. What I'm doing is more supportive. At first, I stepped in there and sort of said, 'Look, this is what you're doing, and this is how you change it.' It doesn't work that way. Now I've learned that, when people come up to me at a party and say, 'He's doing this or I'm doing that, and how can I fix it?' I know now not to offer cookbook advice. I know how to tell them that there are no quick fixes. People get sore at you sometimes for acting like that. They think you've got the answers and that you're just being cute with them.

▲   ▲   ▲

So, in summary, the psychiatric residents appeared to be struggling with most of the same problems as their peers in other specialties: long working hours, financial uncertainty, new knowledge and skills to master quickly, and rapid changes in levels of responsibility not always commensurate with their own developmental progression. In addition, however, there was the constant and more subtle struggle to adapt to a different style of communication with patients and families, to make some inner shifting of gears with respect to emotional comfort with deviant behavior, and perhaps most difficult of all, to assume a rather different posture with patients that depended less on the authoritative mantle of the physician.

BIBLIOGRAPHY

It should be no surprise that by far the largest literature concerns itself with studies and anecdotal reports of stress and coping mechanisms in psychiatric training. There would naturally be a much larger number of faculty members interested in this subject, and the nature of the training itself fosters many developmental problems that stand out in bolder relief in this group of house officers.

The following studies are especially useful in understanding more about the personality substrate of psychiatric residents, the vicissitudes of their training, and the expected changes that occur in them as they progress through their residency. The paper by Fleckles is particularly interesting, having been written by a resident, because it gives a first-hand experience.

Adams PE: Psychiatric residents in blurred roles: Adaptation. Psychosomatics 15:157–159, 1974.
Coryell W: Shifts in attitudes among psychiatric residents: Serial measures over 10 years. American Journal of Psychiatry 144:913–917, 1987.
Fleckles CS: The making of a psychiatrist: The resident's view of the process of his professional development. American Journal of Psychiatry 128:1111–1115, 1972.
Lindy JD, Green BL, Patrick M: The internship: some disquieting findings. American Journal of Psychiatry 137:76–79, 1980.
Scanlan JM: Physician to student: The crisis of psychiatric residency training. American Journal of Psychiatry 128:1107–1110, 1972.
Schneider-Braus, K, Goodwin J: Group supervision for psychiatric residents during pregnancy and lactation. Journal of Psychiatric Education 9:88–98, 1985.
Shershow JC, Savodnik I: Regression in the service of residency education. Archives of General Psychiatry 33:1266–1270, 1976.
Taintor Z, Morphy M, Pearson M: Stress and growth factors in psychiatric residency training. Psychiatric Quarterly 53:162–169, 1981.
Tischler GL: The transition into residency. American Journal of Psychiatry 128:1103–1106, 1972.
Yager J, Hubert D: Stress and coping in psychiatric residents. Psychiatric Opinion 16:21–24, 1979.
Yager J, Langsley DG: The evolving subspecialization of psychiatry: Implications for the profession. American Journal of Psychiatry 144:1461–1465, 1987.

The following group of papers should be helpful in understanding more about the serious, even pathological problems that can occur during training, together with some useful concepts for both prevention and intervention.

Garfinkel PE: Personality, interests, and emotional disturbance in psychiatric residents. American Journal of Psychiatry 138:51–55, 1981.

Russell AT: Emotional problems of residents in psychiatry. American Journal of Psychiatry 132:263–267, 1975.

Waring EM: A preventative approach to emotional illness in psychiatric residents. Psychiatric Quarterly 49:303–315, 1979.

Yager J: A survival guide for psychiatric residents. Archives of General Psychiatry 30:494–498. 1974.

The following group of papers is concerned with trainees who are frankly disturbed and require more attention. The chapter by Scheiber and Henderson, although published in a text on psychiatric training, is quite useful because it surveys the literature across many specialities and many time periods of training.

Kelly WA: Suicide and psychiatric education. American Journal of Psychiatry 130:463–468, 1973.

Russell AT: The emotionally disturbed psychiatric resident. American Journal of Psychiatry 134:59–62, 1977.

Scheiber S, Henderson PB: The Impaired Trainee, in Cohen RL, Dulcan MK (eds): Basic Handbook of Training in Child and Adolescent Psychiatry. Springfield, IL, Charles C Thomas, 1987, pp 247–273.

Just as the transition from student to physician engenders some troubling changes in the trainee, adjustment to the transition from house officer to psychiatrist can be equally disturbing. These two papers describe many of the problems and offer suggestions about anticipatory guidance.

Looney JG: Psychiatrists' transition from training to career: Stress and mastery. American Journal of Psychiatry 137:32–36, 1980.

Dulcan MK: The Transition from Fellow to Child Psychiatrist, in Cohen RL, Dulcan MK (eds): Basic Handbook of Training in Child and Adolescent Psychiatry, Springfield, IL, Charles C Thomas, 1987, pp 321–338.

Chapter 5

NEUROLOGY

Dr. B. is a 30-year-old senior resident in neurology. He is married and has a one-year-old child. His wife is a family practice resident in another hospital in the suburbs. He was the first house officer I interviewed who was dressed in a dark gray business suit, a white buttondown oxford shirt, a paisley tie, and black wing-tip shoes. His hair was cut stylishly. Perhaps he had a perm. I couldn't be sure. He had a resonant voice, and his diction was excellent. His manner was as serious as his appearance. I have seen and heard less impressive figures doing the nightly news.

▼   ▼   ▼

You happen to be interviewing me when I am on my pediatric neurology rotation. I'm an adult neurology resident, but we all get three months on the neurology service at the Children's Hospital because later on you tend to see some kids in your practice and you should have some basic training in the field. I could never do pediatric neurology as a career. I would get dragged down very quickly by some of these devastated little kids you see. If you like kids and have your own or are in the process of having them, it can be very scary looking at some of these patients. Before I had my own, it was different. Now I think, 'There but for the grace of God go I.' There's no guarantee. When you buy a car, they give you a guarantee, but there's none with a child. It always sticks on me.

Somehow, with adults, I can be more scientific and I don't notice the devastation. It's like being in the ER. You don't notice the blood because you're so preoccupied with the patient's blood pressure.

Kids are so vulnerable. If it's an adult with early Alzheimer's or a 65-year-old with Parkinson's or some older person with a bad stroke, you can say that they've had their shot—maybe they had a full life. That kind of philosophy can get you around some of that. After all, 100 years ago, at 65 you were beating the odds. But little kids—I just couldn't take a steady diet of that.

Even some of the young adults I see are tough for me because I still identify with them. I saw a young woman in the ER two days before Christmas. She had two young kids. She complained of being unsteady on her feet. I knew in the first 10 minutes that she had multiple sclerosis. I didn't need any tests, but I told her I wasn't sure. Why ruin her Christmas? I told her to come back in a few weeks, and we'd see how she was doing then. It was clear at that point that she had fairly progressive MS. I confirmed it with the usual tests, and then I had to tell her. She seemed more concerned about the future of her kids than about herself. She was very scared and didn't know which way to turn next.

This is where you get into the problem of informed consent. How could I educate her about MS fast enough and fully enough so she could decide about which of the two or three lousy treatments we have for it and which was the right one for her? She wanted me to tell her what to do. She had no idea and couldn't learn fast enough. Her husband fell apart in front of my eyes. At least in this first meeting, he was useless. I told them it was no emergency. We could take our time and slowly lay out a treatment plan for her to follow.

One thing I do like in the Children's Hospital is that you're not on your own in situations like the one I just described. You cover the unit with a team made up of a pediatric intern, a pediatric resident, and a neurology resident. You're more a consultant on the pediatric cases that have neurology complications. For instance, there are kids with cancer that has spread to the central nervous system, kids with sickle-cell anemia with strokes, kids who have had organ transplants and now have neurologic problems.

The three of us see all the cases together. After we've seen the pediatric cases, then we see mine. My case load is sort of split. There will be a bunch of normal-looking and -acting kids who have strange seizures that we can't explain. The kid may just stare at the ceiling and gurgle. So we bring them into the hospital where they can be observed around the clock. We also have a whole series of very damaged kids who are functioning at low levels. There are lots of esoteric developmental disorders, cerebral palsies, unusual metabolic disorders. Many can't communicate, so you can't even find out how they feel or if anything hurts them.

There are a good many private pediatricians in town who have admitting privileges here, and they send in these very complex cases for what is primarily a neurologic workup and consultation. That's got its pluses because you get to work with a lot of different people and learn their little tricks. What's bad on these complicated cases is that you're working for too many bosses. That's the bottom line. You have the pediatric neurology fellow, the pediatric neurology faculty, the attending pediatrician, consultants from two or three other specialties—it's not a problem until it's a problem. You have five or six groups of people all looking at the kid and trying to explain the problem from their perspective, depending on what particular organ system you happen to like.

The trouble is, you're not sure who the captain of the ship is. The private attending should be, but often he's not, he's just not on top of the case. He's not around enough. And he wants to go along with the consultants, but they don't agree, so the house officer is in the middle. It can be very frustrating. You want somebody to take control, and they won't let you do it. It takes a lot of your time. Eventually, you have to force the attending to make a decision. You sometimes feel like it's the commodities market—you've seen that on TV—with everybody standing up and screaming to get attention. It's like how loud you can scream determines how much influence you can have, instead of a persuasive argument based on some facts.

A lot of unnecessary time is spent by house officers late in the morning or early in the afternoon trying to arrange for special diagnostic studies that were decided on during rounds. Just trying to get a simple test scheduled can be amazingly difficult. You can't leave these to a secretary or even a nurse to do because so often these require some kind of negotiations. They might give you a date that is so far off it's useless. The patient will be gone by then. So if you were head of neuropsychology, I might call you up and say, 'Hey, Cohen, we've got this kid who's got this funny-looking stuff that looks very interesting. We want to send her home Saturday. Can you have somebody take a look at her today or tomorrow?' And you'd send somebody if you like me and it looks interesting enough to bump another patient. No secretary or nurse is going to deal like that. In a way, it's a bit more of the commodities exchange. But this part is not all bad. You often learn something from these negotiations. The other guy will force you to think and to be more specific about what you really want the test for. That means you'll make better referrals in the future and they start trusting and don't ask so many questions.

You can still waste one hell of a lot of time because many of these people are so hard to find. Then you finally get hold of them on Friday and they ask why didn't you call sooner. Then they can say, 'One of my people was sitting around all yesterday morning looking for something to do, and you know, he's got a real interest in that stuff. It's too late now.' You feel like opening a vein.

Some of the afternoon time is good clinical time, though. There are in-house consults to do, and then there is outpatient neurology clinic. Sometimes, I even get some library time. The last thing you do before the end of the day is round with the neurology attending and go over what you've done that day and bring up any questions you have. What I'm describing is here at the Children's Hospital. You have to keep on adjusting to new systems and different hospitals and attendings in this residency. It's one way at Montefiore, and another at the VA, and another at Presbyterian, and so on. Again, you learn a lot from all these people, but you have to keep on shifting gears all the time and mastering new systems of doing things.

A lot of it isn't medicine at all; it's just people. At one of those hospitals, we have incredible hassles with the cardiology and infectious disease people.

If we get a stroke patient in and the carotid arteries in the neck are clear, we just know statistically that 40% of those originate in the heart, that is, the patient has probably thrown off an embolus and it's now lodged somewhere in the brain. Okay, so you call the cardiologist and you ask for an echocardiogram that has some chance of showing whether there is some problem in the heart. The patient has no cardiac history, no cardiac symptoms, and the physical exam of the heart is negative. So they don't want to do the echo. It's not indicated, they say. Negative history — negative physical — no complaints. They say we're wasting their time. But we know about the 40%, and if there is some cardiac problem, it's going to change the management of the patient completely.

You can get the same story from the infectious disease group with the same kind of patient if you suspect that the origin of the embolus was due to pericarditis. We think it looks embolic — and dirty embolic — infected. The patient has a stroke. That's all they know, and they feel it's not their problem. Call them if the patient has signs of infection. This is more of the business of everybody practicing medicine strictly from his or her own viewpoint.

So that's the way the day goes. Some good, some not so hot. Basically, I'm satisfied with the residency from the chairman on down. A training program is easy. It's all or none. You need a good chairman who will let the house officers learn. You need a large, complex patient population. And you need a faculty who can teach you things. You don't want a faculty that just argues about stuff, that doesn't care about teaching and doing neurology, that just likes to argue all the time. That's definitely not our faculty. They're a bunch of free thinkers. They all get along with each other, but each one thinks that the way the others do things is a little crazy. That's all right. You learn more that way. You don't want a bunch of yes men for the chairman to bully around.

If I were the chairman, I'd fire half the secretaries so the other half could get the work done. They could do more work if they didn't have their efforts diffused by all the inept or lazy ones. I can't fathom the attitude of some of these secretaries that work in hospitals. The lack of motivation, the bureaucratic attitude is maddening. We can lose a patient on the floor, and while he's being wheeled out feet first, they're bitching about the paperwork because of a death!

It makes me wonder sometimes how I got into this field. Maybe it was kind of predestined. My father was a doctor, and I was always interested in science and math. I knew I would go into neuro-something because those specialties are more precise. Neuropathology didn't involve enough clinical work. I thought of neurosurgery for a while but I'm not good enough with my hands — too clumsy. I couldn't do that kind of practice anyway. The cases you see are so badly damaged, as the joke goes, that you can consider it a good result in neurosurgery if the patient lives. The average neurosurgeon takes care of a lot of head trauma. You have to go in there and try to do something for people who you know are either going to die or end up in long-term chronic care with a couple of tubes hanging out of them to keep them alive. These surgeons have it rough. They have a few successes they cherish. They also see a lot of low backs that have failed on a lot of treatments—and a lot of chronic pain syndromes in patients who are now so desperate that they'll agree to anything. They just want you to cut it out.

So, by a process of elimination, I ended up in neurology. Not that you get dramatic successes in this field either. You have some patients who stand out in your mind because you have maintained them over a time—the sort of people who could have died several times if you hadn't been there for them. Two, in particular, come to mind as I talk now.

The first one is a guy in his 40s with a fairly severe case of myasthenia gravis. He had an operation to have his thymus gland removed years ago, but they didn't get it all. Then it regrew and he had another procedure, and by now, he's had every type of treatment known for this disease. The outlook for him was not good. Currently, he's looking the best he's been since I started to take care of him. A lot of time and work go into the care of a myasthenia. It's nice to see it work. I took some chances with him. For instance, I had him plasmapheresed, his entire blood volume was washed out. That's controversial, but it worked. He's still slogging along, but he's slogging along at a higher level.

The other patient is a woman who had a stroke. She's had four back operations. She's got terrible hypertension, she's obese, and she had a large neuroma growing on one foot. In addition, she always appeared with an incredible spectrum of symptoms, including headache, insomnia, chest pain, leg pain, belly pain—you name it. After a while, I began to realize how depressed she was. She has responded fairly well to specific treatment of her problems. Just knowing someone was looking after her has alleviated many symptoms.

You really feel like you're doing something with patients like these. If somebody didn't do it, they would be dead by now—or would have killed themselves or done something. You can't just dump these cases. You can't tell them to go to this clinic for this and that clinic for that. Sometimes, the buck stops with you.

▲   ▲   ▲

Several aspects of this interview, and others with neurology house officers, stand out. Again, the "cold bath" aspect of transition from lowly student to responsible physician in a large, busy clinical service is repeatedly emphasized. This is true whether the focus is on the stressful problems of dealing with a complex health-delivery system or whether it is related to the differences in responsibility when one takes over the care of very sick people in large numbers. Dr. B. seemed more harassed by system issues in the hospital where he was serving. Dr. O., a senior-year resident, recalled his early experiences differently:

▼   ▼   ▼

I'll never forget the first assignment I had when I started my training as a first-year neurology resident. I had had one year on a straight internal medicine internship, and there I was, the only house officer for about 25 very sick neurology inpatients. I was it. There was no senior resident, and the attending rounded with me once a day. It was extremely anxiety-provoking. That is what I would call STRESS in terms of both the volume of work and the severity and complexity of the illnesses I was trying to deal with. It got to the point where my self-confidence was so shaken that I began to seek out patients who also had medical illnesses like cardiac or renal problems—I knew something about those and felt more comfortable with those diseases.

It got better as the months rolled by, and by the time I rotated off the service, it was okay. But all in all, it was bad—a cold bath. Too easy to make serious mistakes.

Attendings should be urged to spend more time with the residents early in training. I really did have a terrible time of it those first few months. Also, we should be evaluated by direct observation more often. When I was absolutely at the greenest level, no one saw me do a neurological exam from start to finish—I mean like for the first *six months*, when I desperately needed some feedback on how I was doing.

▲   ▲   ▲

Another two-edged sword that many residents in large, complex medical centers experience stems from circulating among five to eight hospitals during their training experience. The broad exposure to many kinds of patient populations provides diversity of background, but the need to adapt frequently to new systems of operation, new record systems, different nursing staffs, and so on is often experienced as chain-yanking. All of the residents in this group talked about this at length. Dr. B., whose interview is reported at the beginning of this chapter, was certainly no exception.

Dr. U., in describing his experience at the VA Hospital, said,

▼   ▼   ▼

The patients you see at the VA fall into a pattern. First of all, they're 95% men and they're kind of engaging, they're fun if you learn what they want.

There's a kind of camaraderie there. They all share a common experience and they talk a lot among themselves. If you get accepted, they include you in this and you get to know them. Things can get to be very intimate and friendly. Most of them abuse alcohol badly, and most have complications related to smoking, whatever the original diagnosis was. You see a lot of arterial disease, amputees, and strokes—many things that are related to mental status changes—and lots of cancer, especially of the mouth and throat, related to heavy smoking.

I guess the prototype of the VA patient presents you with multiple, interlocking problems: chronic alcoholism, diabetes, vascular disease, and all the neurological complications that go along with abusing alcohol for years with an improper diet. Actually, you can't do much for them. At first, you beat your head against the wall. You try to help them with their social adjustment and give them support to change. You find yourself lecturing and preaching after a while. What you learn is that they are very set in their ways. At first, it's very frustrating because it's in one ear and out the other. You feel you're there to change them, and they're resisting you, like there's a fight between you and they're always winning. It makes you madder and madder.

When you get to talk with their families and learn something about what their lives are like, much of your anger gets dispelled. You start moving away from the strict doctor–patient relationship. You begin to understand that a lot of them will just do the opposite of what the 'doctor's orders' are—or do nothing. Then you still say the same words to them as before because you're supposed to, but it doesn't have the same emotional investment. You no longer expect them to listen—like the paternalistic thing of a father talking to a teenager. You say 'Mr. So and So, here we go again,' and he says, 'Yeah, yeah, yeah.' Sometimes you don't even do that. You just chat about something that's on their mind. It takes quite a while before you understand what that means to them—that a doctor will listen to them and cares about them.

▲   ▲   ▲

By way of contrast, he then went on to describe his experience at the University Hospital:

▼   ▼   ▼

At the University clinic, it's a whole different scene. First, it's strictly doctor–patient, pretty impersonal. A couple of years ago, when I first came here, it was a nice, quiet, smoothly run facility. Now, for some reason, it's being completely renovated and rebuilt. You work in a constant atmosphere of noise and dirt. There is horrendous management—extremely inefficient personnel. It takes forever to get anything done or to get a patient through the system. At the VA, the physical facility is the pits, but the nurses are on top of things. They move the patients through at an incredible rate, yet nobody feels rushed or neglected. And at another hospital we rotate through, it's also very efficient, but at our own University clinic, things just don't run well. You waste a lot of valuable time just sitting around waiting for patients to be 'processed.' I don't know what they're doing with the patients, but I don't see anybody hustling.

If you talk to the people you're supposed to talk to about it, it's 'just another resident complaint—bitch, bitch, bitch,' they say. You never get any concrete answers. Of course, the people you're talking to are the same people who are screwing up the system, so I don't expect a good answer anyway. Now, I've stopped complaining.

▲   ▲   ▲

On balance, one almost always hears the slow, steady progression of these young people through the early stages of panic, growing confidence and strength, and finally, to a sense of mastery. Dr. O., who at the time of his interview had only a few months left to complete his residency, said, "How different it is now when I'm assigned to an inpatient service. I always get in early and make rounds before the attendings get there so I can see the patients first and make the diagnostic and treatment decisions. Then, on rounds with the attending later, if he or she thinks I'm off on the wrong track, we can change things. But I have committed myself and I'm usually right now. That is an enormous boost to your self-confidence."

Another thing that virtually all of the house officers in the medical specialties seemed to value most highly was their ability to collect a case load of their own patients and to run their own continuity clinics. This opportunity to have long-term involvement in the management of a case and to develop stable relationships with patients (and their families) received almost universal approval. This was in distinct contrast to the surgical residents. Dr. B., in his discussion of his patient with myasthenia gravis and his obese patient with multiple disorders, seemed to have no doubts about the importance of his own professional role in the welfare of those individuals.

Patients who might be perceived as unrewarding or frustrating to many types of physicians were not seen in this light by this group. Dr. U. selected this patient from his continuity clinic to tell me about:

▼   ▼   ▼

For instance, there is this 30-year-old woman with chronic headaches. She's been coming a long time. She had so many charts, it would take a week to read them. It's hard to tell how much is self-induced. I had gotten a psychiatric consult on her previously. They recommended treatment, but she couldn't pursue it. She was very reluctant to identify any stresses she was facing, so I brought the family in. Apparently, there's this female neighbor who lives alone and kept dropping in every few days to visit. It turns out she was flirting with the patient's husband. This was a big, big stress for her that she wasn't facing. When I helped her handle the situation, the headaches went down dramatically. I thought we had a real victory here. It had been so bad previously that she would appear at 3 A.M. in the ER asking for Demerol or some other narcotic. Now the headaches are back as bad as ever, and we are back to square one.

That's a common type of patient you see. The symptoms may not be suggestive of any severe disease, but they are very incapacitating. This is her body's way of handling stress. My attending says patients like this have to be handled like any other patient with a chronic intractable disorder. They do okay just knowing that they can come in and that you'll take care of them and that they can see you face-to-face—just so you don't stretch her too much and don't push her toward psychiatric care.

▲   ▲   ▲

However, when the resident's personal and professional resources have been pushed to the limit and when attending supervision does not seem able to resolve the problem, irritation and frustration appear. Dr. O. gave this pithy description of such an outcome:

▼   ▼   ▼

Maybe the most typical example of this type of very frustrating patient is a lady I've been seeing for months in the clinic. She's 33 years old, unmarried, and has two kids. She complains of these weird episodes she calls 'spells.' It's hard to be sure what they are. She does have an abnormal EEG, but she doesn't respond to any form of treatment. I know she feels very sick, and I know there's lots of touble at home. There are many bizarre things going on in her life. She has many gastric complaints and says she can't eat. There is a history of two suicide attempts in the past.

She's just one of these people who pisses me off sometimes and I'm not sure why. I guess it's because I don't know how to handle her. I'm very frustrated. She wants me to stop her spells, but I can't. The most recent spell involved her running out of the house completely naked in the rain and being raped by a mailman. She says she has no memory of this. There have been many other bizarre episodes, and I don't see any light at the end of the tunnel.

My attending tells me just to keep on pursuing the cause of her seizures, which I do, but nothing works. I feel very isolated in terms of trying to get her into some kind of effective treatment. It's easy to be drawn into her problem. She's quite adept at sucking people into her dilemmas. It's hard for me to deal with this objectively. I have to try not to get so frustrated and to keep my distance a little more. I tend to get wrapped up in a lot of nonsense, and then I lose my judgment. Thank God, patients like this are more the exception than the rule.

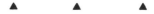

The mind set of the neurologist, in some ways, is that of the careful, meticulous detective who pursues first one clue and then another by a process of deduction until the elusive diagnosis emerges with crystal clarity. Often, neurologists are seen by their colleagues as being obsessional and rigid, and as not having good interpersonal skills. All stereotypes break down, of course. The house officers whom I interviewed certainly did not conform to any stereotype. They did admit, however, that some of their attendings fit that model and were particularly difficult to work with because of their authoritarian rigidity.

Dr. U. was a good example of a budding neurologist who did not fit the stereotype. He said of himself,

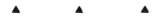

A lot of people tell me I don't conform to the traditional image of the neurologist—you know, this very neat, tight-assed person who's uncommunicative and sort of socially inept outside of professional situations. I don't know how that stereotype developed. It certainly isn't me, and I don't think it describes a lot of people in our program. When I decided to apply for neurology training while I was still in med school, a lot of my classmates kidded me about it. 'Why go into a field where you're not going to help anybody?' they would ask.

It does stick in me a little bit when they tease me, it gets to me. But I don't have any regrets. I think this field has enormous potential for the future. It's a growth field. When you think about how limited our data are, it's a wonder that we help anybody. We're making progress, though, and I want to be involved in that.

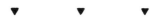

Dr. U., later in his interview, went on to describe his stressful experiences with one of the "neurologic-type" attendings as follows:

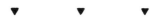

Most people complain bitterly about one of the attendings. He's arrogant, rude, and very abrupt with you. If he doesn't agree with you, he can cut you off right in front of the patient and nurses. If you don't have a lot of confidence in yourself, you can feel wiped out by this. He wants very quick answers, and if you don't have a handle on where he's coming from, you can start taking it personally. Several house officers tried butting heads with him, and that can be the most miserable experience of the whole four years. What I eventually learned when he became vey dogmatic and acted like an asshole was that he's this way with everybody. It's just his style. Once I stopped taking things personally, I started to learn a lot from him. He really does care about the residents. He just can't help the fact that he's hard to be around.

▲   ▲   ▲

Again, it was gratifying to see that, in a large percentage of the house officers, there was this ability to adapt to demands that were often unreasonable and stresses that seemed above and beyond the call of duty, and to retrieve from the experience what was positive and growth-producing.

Admittedly, neurology cannot be classified as one of the high-stress specialties, nor can its residency therefore be placed in that category either. Nevertheless, the stresses that do accompany the expectation of mastering a large body of knowledge, new skills, unreasonable attending physicians, and constant shifting from hospital to hospital cannot be dismissed lightly. Most of these young people seemed to have come into training with a repertoire of coping mechanisms that would help them to extract the most from their training experience.

Chapter 6

DERMATOLOGY

Dr. B. is a 27-year-old second-year resident in dermatology. She is unmarried and a native of a small town in the Midwest. She grew up in a family where both parents were physicians but in other specialties. She has pitch-black hair combed back in a bun and a deep widow's peak. Her bright blue eyes are alive, and she has a ready, dazzling smile. She wore a crisp pale-yellow linen suit, a starched gray blouse, and fragile-looking tan pumps. She was a good talker and needed little prompting to tell her story.

▼   ▼   ▼

When you first get into this residency, you think, oh well, rashes and acne, there's not too much to learn here. As you go along, you realize there is more and more. There really is a great deal to cover. Also, there is a bigger surgical element to derm than most people realize. You have to become expert at those procedures, and you have to learn how to use the laser, especially for port wine hemangiomas and removal of tattoos.

When you're in training, though, you are almost never on your own for surgical procedures, and even in the third year, unless it's something extremely simple. For things like hair transplants or grafts, you are very closely supervised. We have four or five full-time attendings and about a dozen visiting attendings. There's a lot of variation in how they want things done and how they approach problems. You have to learn how they think and you have to work with them in order to get along in the program.

Even inpatient work and outpatient work vary. When you are on outpatient, you tend to move in quickly, look things over, and try to get a fairly rapid result. On inpatient, you want to know more about the whys and wherefores of things, and you do more studies. You are more deliberate in how you proceed because you are often dealing with much more serious problems. On inpatient, you have lots of these blistering diseases, often accompanied by the risk of blindness and a lot of internal malignancies. You have very severe psoriatics who have to come into the hospital because they can't handle the treatment at home with painting themselves all over with tar preparations and using lights and so on. Sometimes you see people with very severe drug reactions whose skin is peeling off almost as if they had third-degree burns.

We rotate through several different hospitals, but you don't necessarily see a lot of different things going from place to place. What you do learn is how to function in private practice, in contrast to the University Hospital. Those are important skills to learn. It's especially important to rotate through these places because we are not allowed to moonlight, so this is our only way of finding out what it's like in the real world. If you don't have this, it can be a very rude awakening.

We also rotate through the Children's Hospital, and I like working with the kids very much. I almost went into pediatrics. The reason I didn't was that, although I do like the kids, I don't like having to do business with the intermediate person, the parent. I like one-on-one work, and that's what you do with adults. It isn't that I mind explaining things to parents. It's that sometimes they want things done and it isn't something a child wants or needs, like removing a little mole from the face at the age of five or six. The child is terrified about what is going on, but the parent has some fantasy about how this is spoiling the child's appearance and you are sort of stuck with it. It can be a no-win situation because, if something bad happens and the kid looks even worse, you can get into a bad bind with the parents. In fact, lots of plastic surgeons and dermatologists won't touch a kid's face for this very reason.

The usual case load in a clinic is 90% acne, warts, dermatitis, or psoriasis. Things can get fairly routine working in the clinic when you see one after another like this. About once a day, you do see something really different or interesting, and then you are likely to call the other residents over to take a look because there isn't all that much new. The seriousness of the disease often doesn't have much to do with how hard it is to take care of the patient. You can have a 17-year-old girl with two little acne lesions on her face and she is very distraught and hard to deal with, and you can have some guy at the VA with pustules all over his face that are weeping and far advanced and he is very casual about the whole thing and does exactly what you tell him to do.

With adolescent girls, it's important to keep your instructions simple and as easy to follow as possible because compliance is an issue. Even when their mothers are with them, you can have compliance problems because they resist the authority of their mothers.

Being on call at night is pretty easy. Most things can be handled by telephone, especially if it is on the inpatient derm service, because you know the patients. If you're on call on the weekends, however, you can plan on coming in a lot because all sorts of things come into the ERs that medical and surgical residents don't recognize and don't know how to deal with. They need a lot of help.

Actually, there are certain kinds of patients I don't like to work with myself. For instance, I don't like hair patients. I think that's probably common because it's such a difficult problem. You are dealing with people's image of themselves. You don't have all that much to help them with. There is one drug that helps some people these days, and of course, there are hair transplants. In fact, to be sure that it's only a congenital hair loss and not a symptom of some serious disease, you really have to work these patients up carefully, and they wonder why. They are very upset about their appearance, and you are doing all these tests.

I guess that reminds me about one of the negatives of this field. You do sometimes get to miss treating the whole patient. You're sort of confined to the skin. You take a lot of kidding about this because sometimes the surgeons and internists look at derm as a fluff field. That really bothered me last year because we took so much kidding from some of the other residents. There is still this myth among other doctors that all there is to derm is 'If it's wet, dry it; if it's dry, wet it; and that's all there is to it.' I'm just beginning to get to the point where it doesn't bother me too much anymore.

Getting a residency in dermatology is very tough. It's a competitive residency, and there are lots more people who want it than there are slots. You have to take electives in medical school and show some aptitude and maybe even do some research in med school and have some papers to show that you mean business. I did both of those things and it helped me get into this program.

It really is pretty good training. I think the only part of this program that I would change if I could is the mandatory research requirement. I guess it's okay for some people, but others can never do it well, and it shouldn't be demanded of them in order for them to get credit for the residency. It's a great source of anxiety and pressure on some people who just can't work that way.

We have no opportunity for electives because of all the mandatory rotations. If research were optional and people were allowed to take electives in other areas, I think it would help. Also, I would allow supervised moonlighting. I wouldn't let it get out of hand. People just don't know enough about what practice is like when they get out of training. Moonlighting is useful not just to make money.

Every three months or so, our attendings fill out evaluations on us, but we never get to see them. We just meet with the chairman once a year in the spring and get feedback. We never get to read the evaluations or discuss them with the people who filled them out. But it's not an atmosphere where you feel like you are constantly being watched and evaluated, so we're pretty comfortable with it.

We are such a small progam, with only nine residents, that everybody knows everybody's business. You are quite intimate, so you have to be extremely careful with how you handle relationships. When you have 50 or 60 house officers and 40 or 50 attendings, you can get some distance between you, but that isn't possible in a department like this. On the whole, I think we are very fortunate in this department because we don't have any poor teachers. Everybody is good. That's great because so much of what you do is one-on-one with the attending. You have to be able to relate to the person and feel comfortable with him. If you are having some trouble, you have to be able to voice it and not feel constrained or made to feel stupid. As I say, I think we are lucky in that regard.

In fact, I guess everybody knows that derm is a low-stress residency and specialty. I'm sure there is a lot of alcohol and drug use in the medical center, but not in our department. These are very conservative people both in training and on the faculty.

That was one of the things that influenced me in choosing this specialty. I come from a pretty square background. Also, I wanted to be able to do a bit of surgery, but I didn't want to go into general surgery and then another fellowship. That's like eight years and a lifestyle that I don't want. The attraction of derm was the ability to work with both adults and kids, to do a bit of surgery, to have a good lifestyle, and at the same time, to be able to use my medical knowledge.

If there was such a thing as director of the residency program in this department, I would like to do that along with clinical practice, but I don't think that exists in dermatology, so I may very well end up in private practice. If you are going into academics these days, you have to do a lot of research, and I doubt if I want to spend my life that way. If you spend your time writing grants, you can't concentrate on educating people and seeing patients. I guess I'll end up in some large hospital on staff seeing patients and teaching, but not in a university setting.

Private practice is not for me. It's you, the secretary, and the nurse. It's just too easy to go to seed intellectually, and you don't have the resources to really take care of very specialized things. It would bother me to have to be referring things all the time to a tertiary center because I couldn't take care of them myself. I want to be able to do that.

▲   ▲   ▲

The house officers whom I interviewed in this specialty seemed defensive about their choice of career. Dr. B. talked about being bothered early in her training because of the kidding she received from others about being in a "fluff field." She protested about the stereotyping of dermatology. For some, the old image of being the doctor who treats venereal disease remained, whereas others talked about their discomfort about being viewed as "cosmetologists" who just fixed up people's appearance when they had little warts or blotches on their faces. Dr. T., a 29-year-old senior resident, described her attitude this way: "What you have ahead of you is a career of seeing people who are usually not very sick and have minor problems. Ninety percent of the practice involves just three or four things that you can recognize immediately, and it may be pretty boring. Perhaps that is why people subspecialize when they get into dermatology, so they can get into more challenging areas. However, you don't do this in most private practices in dermatology. You see the general run-of-the-mill patients, and I guess that can get to be drudgery after a while."

Dr. L., also a senior dermatology resident, said, "You really have to like this specialty to stay in it. If you were a medical student and I were advising you, I would tell you not to go into this field unless you really liked it a lot and thought it was fun. You take a lot of kidding. I mean how can you go to medical school to take care of somebody who has this little spot on his face. You get lots of teasing from the other residents when they see you coming. Like they say, 'There must be a derm code red,' or 'Where are you going—to the DICU (derm ICU)?' You really don't get much respect. It's sort of the Rodney Dangerfield specialty—until they really need you. Then it's different."

These house officers described a level of patient involvement that sometimes involved more responsibility than might be supposed by their colleagues in other specialties. The first manifestations of several life-threatening disorders often appear in the skin as innocuous lesions. It is up to the dermatologist to be acutely aware of these possibilities. The growth of transplant surgery has also opened new doors. It is not unusual for the earliest signs of organ rejection to appear on the skin. Also, there are many dermatological problems that can be associated with pregnancy, so that there are frequent consultation requests from the obstetric service.

Among the most intractable adverse complicatons among diabetics is skin ulcers, particularly in the legs. The house officers encountered so many of these that, in their program, a separate clinic had been established just for diabetic patients.

They had to attend a surgical clinic where they learned to perform skin grafts; to remove moles, birthmarks, and skin cancers; and to use lasers for removing unwanted tattoos.

They spent considerable time on a special rotation in pathology, where they had to learn how to make the clinical correlations between the gross and microscopic pathology and the clinical picture. Dr. L. stated, "This is important for us because most pathologists do not like derm path. There are hundreds and hundreds of obscure diseases that they don't know about, so we have to be able to read these slides often because they can't and tend to avoid them."

The house officers, and sometimes their attendings, were a bit leery about performing cosmetic surgery on a patient's face, especially on a child. No house officer would schedule such a procedure on his or her own and invariably requested the presence of an attending dermatologist, regardless of how senior their status might be in the training program.

Dr. L. stated, "What is still pretty unique about dermatology is that there are really very few full-time attendings. Most preceptors are voluntary private practitioners who come in about half a day a week. Because it is mostly an ambulatory specialty, this works out okay. In our program, we do have some full-time attendings, but they don't precept our clinics. Each has her or his own small specialty clinic, and we rotate through those, but we don't see these attendings for most of our ambulatory work. It isn't terribly useful for learning because these subspecialty clinics don't contain our own patients. You sort of feel like you are tagging along, which is a little tough when you are a third-year resident."

Work with children got mixed reviews, although one of the factors influencing most residents was the opportunity to work with all age groups. Most did not anticipate the problems they would encounter with children and their parents. Dr. L. went on this way: "I enjoyed the children's hospital. Sometimes, the kids are a little scared of the white coat, but you are not doing much to hurt them, and after a while, they start showing off their little warts or their birthmarks, and they almost forget why you are there. Sometimes, the parents can be very upset, especially if a kid has a lot of hair loss or widespread psoriasis because it is so disfiguring. You can't blame the parents for that, and sometimes, they can sort of give you a hard time pressing for answers and rapid cures."

In the final analysis, however, each house officer freely acknowledged that, in addition to the opportunities for high income, minor surgical experience, and exposure to patients of all ages, perhaps the most important attraction of dermatology was the lifestyle it offered. For women who wished to bear and raise young children, the ability to control the time element of practice, its largely ambulatory nature, and the absence of emergencies were especially appealing. Dr. T. summarized things very nicely: "Lifestyle issues were very important for me because I want a family and I don't want medicine to take over my life completely. You can control this practice. You can do it part-time and have parts of your life for other things. I don't have any second thoughts about this. Maybe I would just like to be an affluent housewife and sleep late and have lunch with the girls everyday and play tennis and take care of my baby. Right now, that's very appealing to me. Maybe some day in the future, when my husband is financially secure, that's the way I'll end up. I don't know; maybe I would go crazy after a week of lying around and having fun, but I doubt it. My life isn't tied to medicine."

Dr. L. said, "This is a gentlemen's kind of field. The residency is relatively short, the work isn't hard. The pay is good. The stress is low, and you don't really have to get your hands dirty."

Part II

THE "SURGICAL" SPECIALTIES

The group of medical disciplines known as the *surgical specialties* shares a common approach to the treatment of disease in the sense that their primary treatment modality involves operative intervention either manually or, as technology has advanced, by laser. Although the boundaries between medical and surgical specialties become more blurred as cardiologists perform cardiac catheterizations, dermatologists perform plastic surgery, and gastroenterologists do endoscopies, and as surgeons must be responsible for the overall care of their patients in intensive care units, the general distinctions remain.

This becomes even more evident as one discusses their daily work with medical and surgical house officers. Not only do their responsibilities vary considerably, but what is more striking are those experiences that seem to turn them on about clinical practice. The excitement enjoyed by the resident in internal medicine as he or she problem-solves a difficult diagnostic puzzle stands in sharp relief to the high described by the surgical resident who engages independently in a "bold action" that proves to be life-saving. There really do seem to be important differences between the two groups with respect to their attitudes toward human disease and the most gratifying ways of dealing with it.

For the purposes of this book, I have clustered in this section the specialties of general surgery, obstetrics and gynecology, orthopedic surgery, ophthalmology, otolaryngology (ENT), and neurosurgery.

It is a cliché that every surgeon needs to be a good physician. Nevertheless, as you become acquainted with the house officers in this section, perhaps you will notice what they almost universally described as the "bottom line" in their training: it was most definitely not wielding a stethoscope, thumping on a chest, or writing a prescription for medication.

Chapter 7

GENERAL SURGERY

Dr. O. is a 27-year-old, married third-year resident in general surgery. His wife is a lab technician at the University Hospital. They had met the first week of his surgical internship. He sports one of the few crew cuts I have seen in recent years. He has fine, aquiline features and wears rimless glasses, behind which are a pair of pale blue eyes that miss nothing. Before we moved into the interview proper, he managed some cogent observations about the art on my office walls, the informal arrangement of the furniture, and my medical school textbook on surgery, to him now an amusing antique.

▼   ▼   ▼

Surgery is all I ever wanted to do. There weren't any tough decisions to make along the way. I can't picture anything else for myself. Medicine itself is easy to fall into. Why wouldn't you like it? It's challenging and it's fun. What is it about surgery? I just like making bold moves, fixing things, and seeing the outcome quickly. I'm not sure I'm bright enough to be a really good internist. I don't like the esoteric quality of some parts of medicine. I like to read and be educated, but I can make a decision, and I can act on it quickly. Internists can sit around for hours talking about what they are going to do, but a surgeon has to make a decision rather quickly. You stand there looking at this white belly with no clear-cut markers on it that signal you what to do, and you must decide whether to operate or not to operate.

One of the smartest things I ever did was to take an acting internship during my senior year in med school as a surgical elective—in a Third World country. It's fantastic if you're a med student because all the pathology you see is so exaggerated. You don't see a few bacteria on a smear. You see a whole lung wiped out by tuberculosis. You don't see small, suspicious lesions in the vagina. You see tumors the size of baseballs. It's kind of wild and dramatic, and you have a chance to tackle it almost on your own.

The only bad thing is you don't have the equipment to really study these things. It would be nice to have our technology with those patients. Most of the time, you are just shooting from the hip. You just proceed and treat it anyway. If it doesn't go away, you just find another treatment. You don't culture gonorrhea—you treat it. If it doesn't go away, you find some other cause and treat that. I really feel that six months did fantastic things for me. I had to organize my own time and be responsible for what I was doing. It gives you a great deal of confidence. And you learn not to bitch about small things that go wrong. If you can work under those conditions, you feel spoiled over here.

Right now, I'm just on a general rotation at the University Hospital. The day starts at 5 A.M. There's no time for anything but getting up and running to the hospital. I'm in by 5:30 and round first on the ICU. Then, I see my patients on the floors, both preop and postop. This takes about 90 minutes. Then I meet with the intern and try to give him or her advice or help as needed.

We have to be in the OR and scrub by 7:30. I'm a very time-conscious person. I never run late. I like to stay on schedule, I'm very precise about what I do. I have fairly structured routines. I take my X-ray requisitions to radiology at certain times, and I don't trust anyone else to do it. Same with my lab requests. Things run much smoother that way.

There's a time between 7:30 and 8:30 A.M. when anesthesia is doing their usual monkey business when things slow down, and then it may become difficult to do things at predetermined times. If you've been diligent and got your own work done, you may do some sitting around while you're waiting for the anesthesia people to tell you that they're ready to go. I'm all charged up, and I don't appreciate wasting valuable time like that. Once you start, you turn your beeper off, and you don't pay any attention to the rest of the world—which is very nice.

The goal of every surgery resident is to have as much OR time as possible. At my level, you are given cases based on two priorities: either a gift from the attending, I mean an outright present as a bone, or directly related to your level of development. But some attendings won't give you the bone even if you're ready. It really depends on what she or he thinks of you. There's one attending who never gives any bones. We joke about it. In fact, we've joked about it right in front of him. He laughs but he doesn't change any.

At my level, I might be given recurrent hernias, gall bladders, maybe even up to a liver resection, depending on being in the right place at the right time. A lot of it has to do with making the attending happy: knowing all the lab values, having the films up on the view box and in the right order before you start, being able to answer any questions she or he might have about the patient, being there early and making sure everything is running on schedule. If you have done your homework, and if they think you have been working hard, most attendings will throw you a fair number of bones. You try to get as many things as you can.

It also pays to keep a constant eye on the anesthesiologist. Our relationships with them are generally good, but we see things they don't. They're looking at a bunch of machines and numbers. Sometimes, they have to be jogged, and you ask if maybe some blood shouldn't be started. Or you ask about the patient's urine output. Sometimes, they need waking up because they get a little hypnotized by all that hardware and all the lab values.

I think the residency is dragged out for five years for not very good reasons. It isn't all that hard, and you can learn most of it within a few years. It certainly doesn't take five years to master surgical technique. Most people are ready earlier than they are given credit for. I feel I'm ready to do a large number of cases that I won't be allowed to touch for two years yet.

We spend our evenings rounding again, checking on the cases that were done earlier, and making sure the preop admissions are properly worked up. You try to get out as early as you can. At night, you are doing some of the work that interns do, but they have the responsibility for tracking down every lab value and knowing it. Yet, the next morning, if they don't, you are expected to. You are sort of the backup, sort of the pooper scooper behind the intern, and you had better know the stuff if he or she doesn't. In the OR, though, there is a distinct difference. I can be first assistant on any case with an attending. The intern can't unless we are very short of people or unless it's an emergency.

What time you get home varies a lot. Also, some people tend to tell you that they get home later than they do. If you're observant, what you learn is that most people don't work the hours they tell you they do—nor do they need to. There's no need to be in the hospital until nine or ten every night if you are really organized, diligent, and efficient. There's too much hanging around in the hospital. There's too much of this showing your face and being around in order to earn brownie points. My work style makes it possible for me to get out earlier, and yet sometimes I feel I've been criticized for leaving early even though I've been more efficient.

There is something about sitting around and showing your face at all hours of the night that gets rewarded in the system even though you don't need to be there. The bottom line is that there isn't as much work as people make out. You don't get more than two or three admissions a day. There's no need to turn them into a major performance. Maybe it's true that, once in a while, if you sit around a lot, you might occasionally pick up something that you wouldn't if you hadn't happened to be there. But the unspoken expectation of this does apply a significant amount of stress to the residents because they have to keep such hours even though they may have been on call the night before or they may be on call tomorrow or someone is waiting at home while they sit there waiting for somebody to get a CT scan that they can easily find out about by phone or in the morning.

The business of being on call varies a lot, depending on the hospital and the service. At the VA, for instance, it's every fifth night, and when you're on cardiac surgery, it's every other night. But at the VA, you're the only surgical person in the house, and that can happen to you on the first night of your internship. It did to me. Thank God for that acting internship. I had faced much worse and handled all kinds of emergencies by myself, so the transition was much better for me. At the University Hospital, you're never alone. There are three residents in the house at any one time, but in some places, you are it. Of course, you can always get an attending on the phone if you have questions. A rule you hear is CYA SQUARED (Cover Your Ass and Call Your Attending), but there are some subtleties. You get credit for asking for help when you really should have, but there are some gray areas where people look down on you a bit for asking for help when maybe you should have known better. This is a fine line, and sometimes you don't walk it correctly.

Being on call is not so bad because you can always do more than you think you can. The only time I really felt stretched was on cardiac every other night. There, you begin to get this chronic sleep deprivation, which involves light-headedness and nausea most of the time. Once or twice, I made the mistake of trying to get a cat nap when I would finish around 4:30 or 5:30 A.M. The cardiac fellow isn't needed until about 8:30, and when you see him going to bed for three hours, it doubles your sense of fatigue.

I can't see that this affects your skill level very much as long as you take extra time to think. Anyway, there are almost no situations where you don't have time to consult other people for help even if it is on the phone. So there's very little excuse to stretch yourself beyond your capacity.

I know that a few of the residents smoke pot, but nothing else—no hard drugs. I never see anybody come in unable to do his or her job. I do know there are some people in anesthesiology who are on probation because of substance abuse, but not in surgery. I know a lot of the residents like to party occasionally. You don't do it very often in surgery, so when you do, you blow the doors off, and the next morning, you are not in the best of shape.

There is a lot more good than bad in this residency, but there are a couple of things I'd fix if I could. First, I'd reward people for being efficient and getting their work done well and quickly, and I'd eliminate this foolishness of hanging around. The residents ought to go home when they're finished, have some personal time, and some time to read while they're still wide awake enough to understand what they're reading.

Second, I'd have an understanding with the private attendings that, if you want to be on the staff of a teaching hospital, unless there was a compelling reason, you let the residents do your cases commensurate with their level of skill. The attending would have a crucial role, not just being your first assistant. It would be to help you perfect what you are doing if you are pretty good at it, giving you the fine points and honing your skills. Doing surgery is not all that difficult, but sometimes right in the middle of something, you just get lost and don't know where you are or what to do next. That's where the attending comes in and helps you to get your act together and to understand what comes next.

They have to create the environment for learning. Their influence is pervasive. They can make life miserable for you. If I were the boss, I would try to get some attendings to understand that learning doesn't occur best by living under the gun or the Spanish Inquisition. People don't get more out of the experience by being harassed or intimidated, or by being made to feel inadequate or not up to the task and having their self-confidence broken down. You have to learn how to push people without hazing them. You don't want to take operations away from people for not spit-shining the floor before surgery. You shouldn't hand out punishments by taking away operations. We're here to learn surgery. To learn it, you have to do it. Attendings who want to do all their own surgery should go to a community hospital that doesn't have a residency. If you want to have house officers to do the scut work, see the patients in the ER work up the cases, do most of the postop care, and assist in the OR, you have to give them some things, too. That's part of the bargain.

When you do the surgery yourself, I know you watch that patient like a hawk. Your motivation is different. If you've done a bowel anastomosis, when the fifth day comes around, you are on top of that patient like a blanket. But if someone else has done it, you're less aware of the timetable.

The case I remember best is, of course, one I did myself. There was this fellow on the liver service who ruptured his iliac artery. I happened to be there along with an intern and a medical student. There was no time to call an attending. We knew what it was because of some studies that had been done previously. Within 10 minutes, we had transfused four units of blood and had him in the OR and we saved him. That fits my description of bold action. That kind of thing is fun if you know what's going on.

I suspect I'm going to follow my own advice in the long run. I don't think I'm cut out for teaching and research. I'll probably end up in some community hospital in the midwest with no residency. I don't think I want to be giving my operations away. I want to take care of my own patients.

▲   ▲   ▲

Dr. O. exhibited the characteristics that seem to be common to most of the house officers portrayed in this section. He was very hard-working and action-oriented, possessed a high threshold for physical and emotional discomfort, was disciplined and quite decisive, showed a strongly positive self-image, and almost seemed to enjoy the challenge of high stress. He was not particularly introspective and did not enjoy ruminating over his patients' problems any more than his own.

He seemed willing to do almost any amount of tedious nuts-and-bolts work in order to be given hands-on surgical experience in the operating room.

The case illustration that Dr. O. selected to talk about is a perfect illustration of the "high" stimulated by a clinical emergency in which immediate decision-making and "bold action" is called for, followed by rapid and gratifying positive results. Many of the case illustrations used by house officers in this section are of this type. Conversely, there are many illustrations of cases where the outcome was not a happy one despite the best efforts of everyone involved. The ways of coping with this kind of "low" vary considerably and will be nicely illustrated by other comments as we proceed through the interviews. For the most part, however, they involve the increasing ability of the young physicians to distance themselves emotionally from involvement with the patient as a person and to use a kind of mind set that says, "This is not my fault. I didn't give the patient the disease. I'm not responsible for his or her illness. I did my best and it didn't work out well. It's time to shove on to the next problem."

Because surgery has developed along apprenticeship models, there may be less of a formal curriculum with specific time lines set out for mastering particular skills or bodies of information. This tends to make the process one of happenstance based more on how faculty and attending leaders feel about the way in which a house officer is adjusting, getting along with his or her superiors, and doing his or her job.

One house officer saw it this way:

▼   ▼   ▼

In the surgical specialties, you are there to learn techniques and skills. Knowledge is important, but time at the operating table is everything, and the opportunity to do surgery is the bottom line. This depends entirely on the attending standing across the table from you: if he or she decides to give you the case, you do it; if he or she doesn't, you don't. The criteria are very fuzzy. Sometimes it's based on your level of skill, but very often, it's either based on your personal relationship with the attending or some other things about him or her that you don't even know, or it's a very rich patient, or a very influential patient, or a friend of somebody, and so on. Then there is no way a resident is going to do the case.

There are requirements from the American College of Surgeons about what you are supposed to do—how many cases of each type and so on—during your training, but nobody pays much attention to them. Even if we were reviewed, our chairman is too important and too influential to be questioned. That means that the training you get sometimes does not equate with the standards. That's a shame because most people who go into surgery will work as hard and as long as you require them to. The payback is to get a broad variety of cases to do. In most residencies, the process is too random. If you meet the standards, it's just an accident.

▲   ▲   ▲

In general, there seems to be a sink-or-swim attitude on the part of attending surgeons toward their house officers, perhaps because a career in surgery is seen as such a rigorous and grueling existence that part of training must be a conditioning for the relentless physical and emotional demands of practice. One house officer's introduction to this life came very early in his training. He described it as follows:

▼   ▼   ▼

The pressures of this residency are such that it makes or breaks you. You become fairly hard in a hurry because of all the patient problems and deaths, and also because of the way a lot of the attendings treat you. It starts very early. I remember the first night I was on call as a surgical intern. My first assignment was cardiac surgery, which is an awfully tough place to start. At night, you have to cover not only the cardiac patients but, at that time, the regular floors and the ICU also.

It was my third night out of med school. Now, there are cardiac fellows in the house at night, but then I was completely alone although there were people on call by phone. But I did it. I ran myself ragged. The next day, one of the senior fellows, instead of giving me a small word of encouragement, was quite critical of my management of one of the patients. I don't even remember the details anymore. It was something fairly minor. When my wife picked me up that night after I had been on for 36 hours with no sleep, I was crying silently in the car. I'm not sure she even knew it. I've never cried since although there have been worse days. That was a baptism of fire. You either make it or you don't.

▲   ▲   ▲

It is of more than passing note that this same house officer, now three years later, although happy with his choice of specialty in the sense that he saw it as a good match with his temperament, appeared increasingly frustrated with the current overall image of the medical profession. He had this to say about the subject: "I like the lifestyle. I like accepting responsibility, making rapid decisions, doing procedures, and seeing quick results. I like the level of authority that's involved. I tried internal medicine for a while, but that's not me. I can't think the way those people do, and I can't identify with the personalities in that field. Now that I'm this far along in my career, there's nothing I'd rather do. Obviously, this is the specialty for me. But if I had it to do over again, I wouldn't go into medicine at all. The public reaction to doctors and the status of doctors these days are very depressing. The picture of us as being money grubbing and not interested in patient care galls me. Here I am four years out of med school, and I don't know if I can support my family.

Very few house officers expressed doubt about choosing medicine as a career, although several admitted to occasional mixed feelings when things became hard, fatigue became grinding, finances burdensome, and social life only a memory. For the most part, these proved to be transient episodes of ambivalence, almost always followed by an upswing of mood when exciting new developments were encountered in daily practice or when an attending physician made some positive comments about a particularly tricky piece of diagnosis or a treatment that was well handled.

Always, there were the conflicting yearnings for autonomy and freedom struggling against the needs for "parental" guidance and approval. Clinical rotations were seen as highly desirable if they provided great opportunity for independent action (usually meaning lots of time at the operating table with the accompanying responsibility of being the primary surgeon). At the same time, there was a craving for the guidance of active attendings and frequent feedback that things were going well.

Dr. L., a third-year surgical resident, painted the picture very nicely: "It's wonderful to have your VA rotation for these reasons. When you are there, you are the only surgeon in the house at night. You are on about every fourth night, and if there is any major surgery to do, you and a senior resident do it together. You get an enormous amount of experience. Some people might question the desirability of a couple of trainees doing all that surgery on their own without much supervision. I suppose there is some more risk for the patients, but it's fantastic training. You don't mind staying up all night for that kind of stuff. Contrast that with the University Hospital, where you can get called to the ER at 2 A.M. because somebody has belly pain and the intern can't diagnose a constipated patient with impacted stool and thinks he may have a surgical belly on his hands. That's really a drag. I hate that."

Later on in the same interview, Dr. L. made a special point of talking about how little feedback he was getting from his faculty adviser, about how he is afraid to approach the man directly because he does not know what he will hear, and about how dependent he feels on knowing about his status from his teachers.

Some of these house officers seemed of two minds about their training. Much of what they said was very positive and enthusiastic, but what was negative tended to be strongly so. In addition to their unhappiness with the lack of regular feedback about their progress and the rather haphazard educational plan under which they were being trained, they tended also to complain about their lack of voice in the affairs of the department and about the growing trend toward superspecialization as a force that interfered with their basic development as surgeons.

In regard to the first point, Dr. L., for instance, had this to say:

▼   ▼   ▼

I guess it's just the business of growing up as a competent surgeon and feeling mature while at the same time you are trying to handle difficult attendings who treat you as a child when you are 30. Maybe that last part bugs me the most.

Recently, they have been talking about cutting some of our benefits because of fiscal problems. No one asks us which would be the easiest ones to give up. These stresses are even worse because you are an adult, a husband, a father, and virtually a surgeon, but many people treat you like you're a little kid. That chafes.

The department is very paternalistic. The fathers will take care of all of us, and we are not to ask any questions or worry about anything. That's so inappropriate at our age. Maybe surgery is this way all over. It's sort of the continental style—you know, a few chiefs and all the little underlings.

▲   ▲   ▲

With regard to the second point, that of superspecialization, recall how Dr. O., whose interview opened this chapter, reveled in his experience as a medical student of being immersed in the primary care of very ill patients in a Third World country. He found that very helpful later in adjusting to the demands of a surgical residency, but he sometimes longed for the days when he could take care of very sick patients without the problems of an academic bureaucracy.

The rotations in community hospitals are increasingly valued because the residents see "bread-and-butter" cases there. In the University Hospital, residents do less and less with more complicated, sometimes esoteric problems. Dr. L. stated:

▼   ▼   ▼

More and more is being done by well-trained people in community hospitals. We are getting too specialized. We do a lot of exotic stuff, and this is impacting on our training. When I was on vascular surgery, I did only seven cases in a period of three months. I guess most patients are going elsewhere now. Unless it's something extremely unusual there is almost no reason for a patient to come to a University Hospital anymore. Even things like abdominal aneurisms of the aorta are being done in nonuniversity hospitals. The whole thing has gotten out of kilter. For instance, we have six full-time surgeons on our liver transplant service alone, but there are only about six full-time general surgeons! That tells you something about how the training program works.

▲   ▲   ▲

The extremely advanced and complex nature of many services now being delivered in university hospitals makes junior trainees helpers rather than doers because they may not be seen as having sufficiently sophisticated skills to carry out front-line tasks. One surgical resident said about his stint at the University Hospital:

▼   ▼   ▼

At the end of last year, I was getting very depressed and discouraged because it seemed like no matter how hard I worked, there was too little reward in the operating room. I guess I'll get to feeling better when I'm a senior or chief resident and am getting to do more. Right now, I feel like I'm still doing intern's work for an occasional bone to the dog. There's not much distinction between a junior resident and an intern. The senior house officers don't do much work on the floors—they're busy in the OR and the attendings never do any work on the floors. So you split the work with the interns, which is pretty hard to accept when you are a third- or fourth-year trainee. At one hospital we rotate through, you are up at 5:30 every morning and taking call every third or fourth night. You shouldn't have to do that at this stage of the game. Who the hell wants calls at 3 A.M. after all these years to get permission to hand a patient a Tylenol?

▲   ▲   ▲

There was a tendency on the part of some residents to see the training as being unnecessarily prolonged for these reasons. Sometimes, the residents viewed themselves as being kept in a state of professional immaturity, a kind of hibernation from which they would be turned loose after five or six years, when, in fact, surgical skills can be learned more rapidly than that.

When all was said and done, however, most of them would not have wanted to do anything else. They saw surgery almost as a calling, good only for certain kinds of people with certain interests and talents. They viewed the sleep deprivation, the fatigue, the not infrequent harassment from attendings, the separation from the family, and their uncertain professional futures as burdens to be borne—and sometimes to be complained about. But most seemed driven to do what they were doing.

As Dr. O. said, "Being on call is not so bad because you can always do more than you think you can."

BIBLIOGRAPHY

Linn DS, Zeppa R: Does surgery attract students who are more resistant to stress? Annals of Surgery 200:638, 1984.

Chapter 8

OBSTETRICS AND GYNECOLOGY

Dr. R. is a first year resident in obstetrics and gynecology. He is 28 years old, is married, and has two small children. His wife is an M.B.A. working in the trust department of a large bank. He insisted on coming to my office even though he was currently on a surgical schedule and I offered to meet him at his hospital, which is located five long blocks away. He was dressed casually in a golf sweater, scuffed suede shoes, and tan cords. He spoke rapidly and had little patience with the small talk that I had found useful as a warm-up or "connecting" exercise at the opening of an interview with a young colleague who might be a bit wary of chatting with a psychiatrist she or he was meeting for the first time. Dr. R. would have none of that. He was all business. It was 4 P.M., and I wondered if that wasn't a very busy time of day for him.

▼　　　▼　　　▼

No, not usually that busy a time if you're efficient. I'm on what's called the private GYN service now. Mostly, this involves taking care of the daily case load of the private docs who have admitting privileges: working up the patients as they come into the hospital, assisting during the surgery, and managing the postoperative care. This year, I don't get to do much surgery on my own. Later on in the training, you get assigned to the clinic GYN service, which is largely run by the residents with faculty backup. Then you're the primary surgeon on most cases. This service is really not a demanding one. They don't expect that much of you.

The toughest part of this year for me is night call, which is about every fourth night. That means the emergency room, where a lot of the time you are on your own. You can usually get hold of a senior resident if you need help, but sometimes they're in the OR and you just have to wing it. Things are very busy there until about 10 P.M. The most important decisions you make have to do with who has to be admitted then and where, and who can be referred to one of the outpatient clinics or back to her private doc. There's lots of nonspecific pelvic pain, people with unexplained vaginal bleeding, or sometimes you see women who are being treated as outpatients on the oncology service and they're having bad side effects from their chemotherapy.

There is the usual parade of teenagers who are afraid they're pregnant and—I know this is hard to believe, but a couple of nights ago I saw this 15-year-old black girl who was complaining of infertility! She said most of her friends were pregnant and she wasn't. Could I find out what was wrong with her? There was some kind of peer pressure in her group to be pregnant. It was like a membership club.

Things slack off there after 10, but then you're on backup call for the OR in case they have two surgical emergencies at once and you have to scrub in. Even though we may be pretty tired at that point, nobody ever bitches. We want to be called in. The name of the game is to get hands-on experience in the OR. That's everything.

You asked me about a typical day, and somehow I got started with night call because that's the hardest part of the day. I'm usually up at 5:30 A.M. I must make an early start. On this service, it's you and the attending. There's very little help from the senior residents. So I have to get a lot of things done before surgery starts at 7:30 A.M. My wife makes a later start than I do, so she manages the kids mostly in the morning and I do more at night if I'm home. I'm in the hospital by 6:15. This is one of my favorite times of the day because I make rounds alone. I see every patient, make the necessary decisions on the postop patients, and write the orders. The attendings come in later and round by themselves. They can change things, of course, but they seldom do. They're really concerned about liability suits, and they know that if they change an order, they'd better have a damn good reason for it if something should happen to go wrong later. When they do change something, we talk about it later, and I learn a good bit from that.

What I love about those early-morning rounds is that I must commit myself first, before the attending says anything. If you make rounds with a senior person, you're naturally always deferring to him or her. Or even if you come right out and take a position on something, in the discussion that follows, you often get talked out of it. This way, you make a clinical decision, and the burden is on the attending if he or she wants to change it. That's optimal for my type of personality. I don't find it stressful to be on my own. Decision making is what this field is all about.

I don't want to blow this up into some big deal. Most postop care is pretty cut and dried. There aren't that many big decisions. The major differences I have with attendings is why some people are operated on in the first place. See, I have no control over why the patient is admitted to the hospital. If she consents to the procedure and the attending wants to do it, then it's a given. All these decisions are made by the time you see the patient, and you have no input. You may object to the indications for surgery, but you're obligated to assist. This is when most of the house officers have trouble. We talk about it among ourselves. We're disturbed about it, but we feel impotent. What I'm saying is that the things you have the most conflict over, you have the least control over. The patient may consent out of exasperation with her illness, but you know lots of these procedures are not going to benefit the patient, unless it's in a mental sense — like they're doing something just to do something. But you have to live with it. You can't say anything to the patient.

Probably the most common reason for this kind of thing in GYN is chronic pelvic pain. No one understands what's going on. So the surgery is done as a kind of therapeutic trial. I have real trouble with that when you go in to work up the patient the day before and there are very obvious underlying psychiatric problems. It's almost like the attending is doing the surgery so he or she can refer the patient to a psychiatrist afterward when no organic reason has been found for the symptoms.

Or you operate and find lots of adhesions from previous surgery. Now, adhesions are caused by inflammation or from violating the peritoneal space. What sense does it make to violate the space again to break up adhesions when you're going to cause more adhesions? Maybe they're hoping the new adhesions won't cause as much pain. You see some women coming in three or four times for this when you know that, most of the time, you're just multiplying their problems.

This is what I have the most trouble with. I don't see these same women months or years later. Maybe it helps some of them. I see others coming back, though. I admit I don't have the big picture. Maybe there is some long-range benefit for some. Also, I don't have to live with these women year in and year out. Maybe if I were in the attending's shoes, I'd do the same thing out of desperation. There are about 30 or so private attendings here, and some do this kind of thing a lot more than others. Because surgical assignments get passed down the line by the senior residents, the more junior you are, the more you have to scrub with these guys because no one wants to do it. Also, these turn out to be the most difficult patients to deal with personally, and so are their attendings. Sometimes, the house officers or the head nurses will discuss psychiatric referral with the attendings, and they will listen. You couldn't see some of these women in your office day in and day out without going bonkers yourself.

Strangely enough, it isn't the patient with persistent complaints without organic pathology who gives me the most trouble. It's the extremely demanding patient who acts like the world owes her a living, the ones who expect special attention. You might think it is always Mrs. Gotrocks who acts like this, but that's not true. Money seems to have nothing to do with it. They come in with a chip on their shoulder. Some are clinic patients and some are private. If they don't get what they think is coming to them, they seem to hold the threat of litigation over your head. You feel like you're walking on ice chips or egg shells. When I'm put on the defensive early, I seem to have more trouble with people. I'm not very good at defusing volatile situations because I get angry and lose control of what's going on. If someone is in pain or having trouble coping, I can be more sympathetic, I can give them more.

A lot of clinic patients are incredibly demanding. They seem antagonistic because they are on medical assistance. They use our emergency room like an outpatient clinic. Routine blood work that might cost 35–40 dollars in a clinic is going to cost 75–125 dollars in the ER, at three o'clock in the afternoon. How much surgery you get to do yourself depends on the attending and how much she or he trusts you. Sometimes, you've held retractors for five hours for one private doc after another without doing much. But they all have little tricks you can pick up by watching carefully. Each one comes in fresh and rested, but you may have been up much of the night and you've had no lunch. It takes discipline. After you've written all the postop orders in the recovery room, you go back to the floor and check your surgery assignments for the next morning. The senior resident decides what you get, and if you're low man, like I am, it's the leftovers. I guess if I have any complaint about this residency, it's the rigid hierarchical system between the years. The borders and territories are marked off by way of privileges and power. Sometimes, you offer to pitch in and help with something, and instead of being rewarded for being a good team player, you're scolded for stepping on somebody's toes.

Anyway, after you've worked up your new patients for the next morning and taken care of any little problems that have come up, you're free to sign out if you're not on night call. Sometimes I'm done by 4 P.M. unless there's an emergency in the OR and they need me. Mostly, the senior residents grab those. As I said, the name of the game is experience. That's the gravy for all the routine work you do. When I'm a senior resident, I'll get the goodies. Maybe it's not such a bad system.

Because I'm finished most days before my wife, I pick up the kids. One is in day care and the baby is with my mother. I start dinner and play with the kids. My wife gets home between 6:30 and 7 P.M. We have a late dinner, and I put the kids to bed while she cleans up. Then we just read or watch TV before bed. We have almost no social life. There's just no time between our schedules, the kids, household chores, and so on. I've got over three years of this yet, so we have to take it easy on the money side, too, with a couple of kids. They really add to the stress and pressure. They're wonderful, but our lives would certainly be a lot simpler without them.

My wife is kind of uptight about the situation. She's going through the typical career-mother syndrome. I think she's more upset than the kids are when she's late or can't follow through on something we promised the three-year-old we would do. This happens pretty often with our schedules. I think the kids are fine, and I try to tell her so and support her, but I don't think it has much impact. She imagines great harm coming to them. She's one of those people where the more you talk, the more inflamed the issue becomes. So I try to soft-pedal it. It's like a sore. If you don't pick at it, it'll probably heal.

We didn't really intend to have two kids this early. The baby is only six months old and just sort of happened. My wife had him right here in this hospital, which was quite an experience for me. Although they let me in the delivery room, they made me sit up at her head like all the fathers do; I had to stay out of the field. The nurses even made me wear the scrub suit that fathers wear instead of the regular blues. You're very vigilant. You know all the things that can go wrong, and you want to know everything that's going on. There were some ominous signs on the fetal monitor, and there was tension in the labor room. The attending was starting to get anxious. I knew what was going on, and my wife was getting very upset with me because I wasn't telling her the truth. It all turned out OK in the end, although the baby didn't look so great when he came out and it took about 10 mintues for him to pink up. In a way, it was good. You're not so short with the patients and their husbands when you realize what they're going through.

Before I started my residency, I always thought of myself as an obstetrician, but that's undergone a major change. I found my obstetric rotation a whole other world. It's like working on an ICU but with patients who don't have any disease! There's a very high level of tension. You've got a very experienced nursing staff, and you're highly dependent on them. As a house officer, you walk around always feeling that something is about to break. I felt like I was walking on the edge of disaster all the time, especially in the beginning. After a while, you learn which people to read. It's like the sheep watching the birds when there's a predator around. When you see certain nurses start running, you know there's an impending disaster. When you've been there a while, you learn which birds to watch.

That experience caused me to do a one-eighty. Now I see obstetrics as a kind of necessary evil that I'll have to do to earn a living. But I don't like the atmosphere. You don't feel in control. You can't relax. So much is done to cover your butt. There's so much litigation. As a junior house officer, I was always being second-guessed by the senior people. Everybody was so afraid of something going wrong. The procedures in an uncomplicated delivery are fun. The field itself isn't. I didn't have any bad outcomes during my six weeks on the labor suite, but one of the other house officers wasn't so lucky. He missed picking up a breech presentation and, worse yet, tried to induce labor. You just don't do that on a breech. Luckily, it was caught before things went really bad, but the maximum of guilt was extracted from him by the senior resident and the nurses.

Now that I think about it, I don't know what the big appeal of OB was. I'm much more interested in surgery, which is basically what GYN is. In med school, I was very much disenchanted with internal medicine and the other medical specialties. You're so limited in what you can do. The perceived benefits are so much less than in surgery. Most patients come back in six weeks, and they look good. There's more direct feedback, and you don't have this big collection of chronic patients with limited results who come to see you forever. That kind of life would bore me to tears.

▲   ▲   ▲

The reader will quickly recognize many common themes that run through these surgical subspecialties, particularly those that had to do with the importance of hands-on operating time and the whole issue of how decisions were made about when a particular house officer was ready to carry out a given procedure. The "bone to the dog" or "gift" orientation of surgical attendings, which was perceived by many residents, was a pervasive subject. There is no need to belabor it further.

Rather, let's consider some of the issues that may be more specific to obstetrics and gynecology. In some ways, these two specialties have been lumped together because they share a common organ system within the female body. It is true that they are both largely surgical specialties and that they involve the care of the female reproductive system, in both its normal and its diseased states.

There are, however, many differences both in approach and in practice. The joys of caring for the normal, radiant gravid woman and of bringing new life into the world have been soured by the growing societal expectations of magical interventions on the part of the medical profession and by the litigious nature of everyday life in medical practice. Young parents want and expect healthy, normal offspring. If, in any way, the obstetrician is perceived as contributing to the production of an abnormal baby, a suit charging negligence can be expected to follow shortly.

Dr. R., toward the end of his interview, spelled out the 180-degree turn that ensued in his own thinking and planning as he was exposed to the high-tension quality of obstetrical practice in the 1980s.

Another resident described in graphic detail the contrast he experienced between the gratifications of gynecological practice versus what he portrayed as the "craziness" of modern obstetrics:

▼   ▼   ▼

There's a follow-up patient we see in the postpartum clinic. I've gotten to the point where I don't want to give her the time of day anymore. We had to do some electronic fetal monitoring when she was in labor because she was having a lot of trouble getting the baby through the birth canal. All that involves is placing this tiny spiral electrode in the fetus's scalp when the mother's cervix is dilated enough. It's hardly more than breaking the skin.

Then you hook the head up to a monitor that checks the pattern of the baby's heartbeat. It's really a safety measure and lets you know if the baby is in real distress, in which case you might want to do a cesarean section and get the baby out of there before there is any brain damage from excessive pressure on the head or from not enough oxygen getting through. It's a harmless procedure [fetal monitoring]. Well, this lady has gone bonkers over this little pinprick left in the baby's scalp. She says the baby looks funny to her and that there is some trouble with his eyes; she thinks maybe he'll be blind as a result of this! We're not taking care of the baby. A pediatrician is doing that, and he has reassured her that everything is fine with the baby, but that doesn't stop her from badgering us about it. She has my name, and she knows I was the resident on the case. Every time she sees me in the hallway, she has 20 questions about what was wrong and why we used the monitor. There really is no problem. Everything turned out just fine. She's the kind of person who could drive me out of this field.

You look at her, and then you go up to the oncology service where these really terrific women are fighting for their lives going from surgery to chemotherapy to radiation, their whole existence and family life thrown into turmoil, and you look at their husbands walking slowly up and down with them pushing the IV stand in front of them so the medication can keep going while they walk. Then you say to yourself that maybe you'll stick it out in spite of the pest with her obsession about fetal monitoring.

▲   ▲   ▲

It is with **patients** such as the mother of this fetal-monitored baby that the deficiencies in surgical training stand out in boldest relief. Many residents complained of situations like this. It was immediately evident that there was nothing in their faculty teaching or supervision that ever caused them to stop and ask themselves whether there might be a difference between the overt and the covert questions confronting them. This house officer had no tools in his diagnostic repertoire that might assist him in understanding what this distraught mother was really upset about and how he might, therefore, intervene.

But it is in the nature of the personality makeup of most practitioners of the surgical specialties to view such patients as unrealistically demanding, weak, troublesome, and very unrewarding. Quick, clean results are prized beyond all else. And yet, a house officer may be perfectly capable of being turned on by a special case of a very seriously ill, vulnerable patient whom he or she views as requiring special attention, in contrast to the "routine" problems confronted every day (and, perhaps, regard-less of their gravity). Dr. D., a 27-year-old third-year resident, described such a case to me as follows:

▼   ▼   ▼

For instance, I now have a 14-year-old girl on the floor who really stands out in my mind as someone I must pay special attention to over the next several weeks. Suddenly, three days ago, she discovered this mass protrud-ing out of her vagina. Her mother went bananas. The family doctor referred her here. It almost certainly is what's called a botryoid sarcoma. These are usually fatal within one year. She's an only child. She's terrified and her mother is hysterical. Today, the kid is going through all the studies to deter-mine the actual size and spread of this.

For some reason, my heart goes out to this girl. I feel an extra respon-sibility to explain things to her and to simplify things so she understands what's being done and why. The attendings have certainly not acted any differently toward her and her family than they have with all the other patients. It's been business as usual—very terse, very brief. All I can do is use my special knowledge of gynecology to help her.

I'm not an especially talkative or articulate person myself. This isn't my bag, but I'll try. She'll be here for weeks. She needs one person to look to for an understanding of what's going on. If I were the attending, I would take her by the hand and lead her gently; I'd tell her everything so she would see the logic of what's being done for her. There aren't any facts and figures to give her. The condition is too uncommon.

Wait until she finds out that she will have to have a total hysterectomy. She may even need to have all of her pelvic organs removed and have a colostomy. It can be very disfiguring. My biggest fear is that she'll panic and want to leave the hospital before she gets enough treatment. Maybe I can build up enough trust with her to help her go through these procedures.

She's somewhat unusual on this floor. Most of the patients are a good bit older, in their 50s and 60s. There are lots of women with ovarian cancer who have had surgery and now come back every few weeks for chemotherapy. It's interesting but not very exciting to work with them. They seem resigned to their fate. There's a lot of depression in this group. Things are fairly predictable with them—not too many surprises. I like it more when some-thing different happens.

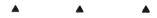

Perhaps the above is an illustration of the fact that young physicians need the exotic and the dramatic in order to perceive something "different" in a patient or in a disorder. They need the discernment of their teachers to see what is different in every situation and to be rewarded by dealing with it in an individualized manner.

Unfortunately, the modeling, by which much teaching at this level occurs, is more often that of the reserved, uncommunicative, even forbidding surgeon. Dr. D., who was a house officer on the oncology GYN service, described his teachers as follows:

▼   ▼   ▼

When you come right down to it, there's not a lot of communication between the attendings and the patients and their families either. It's just not a high priority for these doctors. Nobody's really hiding anything, but there is a big gap between what the patients find out and what the attending is doing. The social workers on the floor complain about this, but nothing much happens. The doctors make it clear that it isn't something they want to spend their time on. They just don't like talking to families and explaining what's going on. So most of it is left to the nurses and social workers, which is not the most satisfactory thing.

It's interesting to watch the house officers model themselves after the attendings. You can see it happening. If it isn't a priority for the attending to spend time explaining things, then the house officer acts the same way. I guess it's the skills that are a real challenge. On the other hand, most of these women with ovarian cancer have a lot of problems in common. Ovarian cancer is a bad disease because it's usually so silent and tends to spread before it is picked up on routine pelvic exams. So it's very hard to get all the tumor surgically, and many of them don't respond to chemotherapy. The two-year survival rate if the tumor has spread to any part of the bowel is only about 10%–12%. That means that most of these women are going through very strenuous and unpleasant treatment, and yet the chances of their being around a few years from now are not very good.

▲   ▲   ▲

Dr. D. felt compassion for the patients but, perhaps, just as much for his superiors, who had to face dying women every day and had finally withdrawn themselves emotionally from the patients and the families. Dr. D. had discovered that he was not properly wired up for the life of GYN oncologist. He said very emphatically, "I'm already learning that I'm not the right kind of personality for this. Maybe I can't distance myself from it and be impersonal enough to handle this kind of life year in and year out. Also, to be very good at this, you have to be extremely demanding on the staff, especially in the OR, to get things done exactly the way you want them and not be too concerned about sensitivities. These attendings are very good at both things: remaining impersonal and being absolute dictators concerning procedures. The nurses make jokes about them behind their backs, but you can tell they respect them."

Dr. D. described his own interaction with these attendings as stressful, impersonal, and akin to the hazing process we have already heard so much about, as follows:

▼   ▼   ▼

Attending rounds start late in the afternoon. We all meet in the ICU to see the most critical patients first. Then we go to the floor and see every patient. We go over the charts first. It seems that no matter how hard you've worked to get every detail into the chart and to master the information yourself, they always come up with something you never heard of—something we should know but don't. This is a very stressful time every day. You're trying to look your best and come up with the right answers. It gets to be kind of a game where they're trying to trip us up. [He laughs.] I'm not convinced it leads to any useful learning on our part. It's kind of like a hazing process or a one-upmanship thing.

Maybe what we learn out of it is to be compulsive, and I guess that's important. It puts the onus on us to get all the details and to make some sense out of them. It really keeps us on our toes, and that's better for the patients. Basically, I don't object, although sometimes it can be very painful.

▲   ▲   ▲

So young house officers in obstetrics and gynecology have some difficult career decisions to make. If they aim their sights in the direction of the conventional practice of obstetrics, they may come to see that rather physically grueling existence as one of merely "receiving babies" without being able to use much of their excellent medical and surgical training. If they decide to focus on the serious, life-threatening disorders seen in gynecology, they know that they must develop into superb surgical technicians, but that their emotional life may become totally isolated from their practice if they are to survive psychologically.

At the same time, as they survey the obstetric landscape, they see many alternative systems of health care developing that take many prospective pregnant patients out of their practice. The emergence of out-of-hospital birthing centers and home delivery programs run by nurse-midwives is a serious threat to the economic survival of obstetricians. Often, in good conscience, they must openly object to these developments because they feel the procedures are not safe, but in doing so, their motives are suspect.

One house officer put it this way:

▼   ▼   ▼

Things can go bad faster in obstetrics than in any other specialty. You can have a perfectly healthy woman who will become preeclamptic, develop pulmonary edema, go into seizures, and die—all within six hours. These are the kinds of cases I want to try to do something about.

This is why the big trend toward home deliveries and out-of-hospital birthing centers is wrong and stupid. It's the last legal kind of child abuse. Maybe only 1 in 100 deliveries gets into trouble. But the problem is that you can't predict which ones they will be. I've seen kids die in 20 minutes from what seemed to be a normal state—and that's in the hospital!

You just can't handle these problems outside the hospital. I can see how parents develop these attitudes. They don't see the bad experiences. They talk to their friends who have had normal babies. Then you expect your baby is going to be normal, not that 1 in 100. But when you start thinking about it, that's a lot of babies.

▲   ▲   ▲

Many young house officers have opted to move in the direction of high-technology obstetrics as a reasonable compromise between the demanding world of GYN oncology and the rather boring existence of the traditional obstetrician. This permits them to use all of their medical and surgical background as they perform cesarean sections and intervene surgically in the serious problems of ectopic pregnancies while, at the same time, caring for the serious medical problems of the high-risk pregnant woman who comes to the labor suite with diabetes, hypertension, or toxemia.

Chapter 9

NEUROSURGERY

Dr. F. is a 27-year-old, unmarried, second-year resident in neurosurgery. He is the second of six children. His father is a "medical architect" specializing in hospitals and medical office buildings. He is from the Southwest, where he went to college and medical school. He carries himself like a West Point cadet, erect and with a walk that suggests someone was counting cadence quietly in his ear. Scrub suits never fit well, but somehow, his did, despite his wiry physique. The corners of his mouth turned up ever so slightly, so that it was difficult to be sure when he was smiling. It is a Mona Lisa mouth. During the session, he volunteered almost nothing. There was no reaching out. I had to come to him. Self-containment most nearly describes his mode of interpersonal transaction. He was not a subject for an inexperienced interviewer. Several times, as we talked, I pictured him 35 or 40 years from now, a crusty curmudgeon, chewing out house officers for minor transgressions—with relish.

▼   ▼   ▼

Training in neurosurgery means a seven-year commitment after medical school. The entire time is pretty structured, so you know what's coming. The first year is straight general surgery. That's so you develop the basic surgical skills and get very comfortable in the atmosphere of the OR. The second, fourth, and seventh years are all straight neurosurgery divided between adults and children in different hospitals. The third year, you get a mix of neuroradiology, neuropathology, and neurology. The fifth year is spent in basic research, and the sixth year, you can either do more research if you want to or spend some time learning how they do neurosurgery in another university center somewhere. That's the seven years, and I'm only in the second one. But I love it.

In some of the hospitals we rotate through, you're the only resident there at any one time—like the VA. So, for those three months, you're on call every night. That's why it's good to have the program broken up the way it is. In some of those middle years, you have the time to think and read and do some writing, which is very important if you want to launch an academic career. If you wait seven years to start turning out original papers, it's too late to get started. You're approaching your middle 30s by then, and there are plenty of younger guys who've gotten into the academic pipeline ahead of you.

A typical day varies enormously, depending on whether it's one of the clinical years or not. During a clinical year, your day starts at 5 A.M. because you must round on every patient on the floor, see all the neurosurgical patients in the ICUs, write your progress notes on the charts, and go through morning report with the attending and the senior resident all by 7:30, when you have to be in the OR, scrubbed and ready for the first procedure of the day.

If you're on something like neuropathology, that's like a day at the beach because you're not in until 8 A.M., and the day is spent reviewing slides from yesterday's surgery, or examining gross surgical specimens. Then you write reports on these and meet with the neuropathology attending to go over your findings, and he or she either corrects anything wrong or signs off on it. These are good teaching sessions because they're one-on-one with very experienced faculty. Also, when you're in these nonclinical years, there's no night call. These are very low-stress times.

In many ways, the business of night call is the hardest part of the training. It's not getting up so early. Surgeons love that. It isn't standing on your feet most of the day for these three- and four-hour procedures. You're doing what you really want to do. It isn't seeing all the patients and admitting and working up so many patients. It's generally being on call most of the time. It's either every other night, or if you're the only resident on that rotation, then it's every night for several months. Part of it is that this is such a big trauma center. You get as many patients some nights as can be transferred at one time.

When you're on, theoretically, you can call the chief resident or the attending who are not physically in the hospital. But it gets to be a matter of pride. You don't want to do it. You want to deal with it all by yourself. It's also a good idea to take it easy on the chief resident who is on call every night that year and doesn't even get home on the average night before 10:00 or 10:30. You really don't want to call him or her. There's something about handling it all by yourself that gives you a good feeling. I don't know how many neurosurgical residents you've interviewed so far, but you'll find we have very big egos.

I seem to attract heavy traffic when I'm on call. I've sort of gotten this image in the hospital. When somebody looks at the schedule and they see I'm on, they say, 'Oh, oh, it's going to be a wild night.' It's gotten to the point where I don't even plan to go to bed. Then you start feeling tired. I just plan to stay up all night, and it works out that way.

A good example happened a few weeks ago. Things were reasonably quiet until about 11 P.M. Then this suicide attempt came into the ER. He had tried to shoot himself in the head but hit himself in the face instead. Apparently, the bullet passed along the base of his skull, but we couldn't be sure whether he had grazed the base of his brain or not because of all the bone damage and bleeding. I got the general surgical resident and the maxillofacial resident to see him, too, in order to play safe. As far as I could tell, there didn't seem to be any significant brain damage.

By this time, it was about 2:30 A.M., and the phone rang from one of the suburban hospitals. They were sending in two trauma patients from the same car accident. One had a major neck injury with possibly a severed spinal cord, and the other was thought to be a closed-head injury. I tried to suggest that it might be a good idea to send only one to us and send the other one to another hospital because I was on alone and those patients sounded as if they would need a lot of immediate attention, but they wouldn't have any of it. They said it had been a very bad night out there, and they had already transferred several trauma cases to nearby hospitals. So I was it.

Here I was with this gunshot wound that had to be watched carefully—a patient with a possible severed cord, and for him you have to put these tongs in the skull and put the neck in traction with weights to take the pressure off the cord—and a closed-head injury with an unknown amount of brain damage. I was running between the CT scanner, where we were trying to reduce the dislocation of the patient's cervical vertebrae—I had to be there because when a patient like that is in the scanner, you have to detach him from the traction apparatus, so I had to pull on the tongs myself while supporting his neck manually. No one else would touch the tongs. I wouldn't let them anyway. And then I would dash and see the other two patients quickly to make sure their status wasn't deteriorating. The neck patient took enormous time because it takes so long to put the tongs in and reduce the dislocation.

I was really worried about the head injury, although he didn't appear to be in very bad shape. You can't tell with those. You get this silent bleeding, and suddenly, because of the pressure, their brain stem can herniate into the spinal canal, and it's curtains when that happens.

Nevertheless, I felt I was on top of all this and that the patients' care was very good when two things happened. First, the scanner in the University Hospital went down, and I had to transport the neck patient down the hill to another hospital, maintaining hand traction on the tongs myself while I got him into their scanner. While I was down there, the charge nurse on the neurosurgery unit at the University Hospital called to tell me that a patient on the floor had suddenly become cold and clammy and his blood pressure was dropping. There was no way I could let go of those tongs, and by this time, it was almost 5 A.M. and I knew the other residents would be in any moment, so I told her to hang on for a few minutes and keep the patient stabilized until somebody came. One of the residents did show up a few minutes later and took over, so it was OK.

By that time, I had to go wash up and start my own rounds so I could be ready for the OR by 7:30 A.M. Although that night was a bit unusual because of so many things happening at once, most of the nights are pretty bad in the sense that we're very busy. Then, you're up all day the next day in the OR because there are three rooms going and only three residents to assist. You're tired, but I don't think the quality of my clinical judgment or my work goes down. What happens is that it takes me much longer to figure out the right thing to do or the next steps. In the end, I do the right thing, but there is a slowing down of all of the mental processes. You just don't work at the same speed. You'll think of something and think of it again and then run it through your mind the third time, and finally, you'll say, 'Why am I thinking of this so much? I was right in the first place.' You'll sit there writing orders and ask yourself what you want to know about this patient tomorrow morning, and suddenly it will come to you that this patient has seizures and is on an anticonvulsant agent and it's been several days since you checked the blood level of the drug, so you write the order. When you're wide awake, that would have taken five seconds.

Some residents, when they are like this, tend to get very snappish with the nurses. I don't. I get very complacent and quiet because I know it's going to take me a lot longer and involve a lot more energy to get something done.

The business of handling death and dying in neurosurgery is rather different, I think. You get used to it pretty quickly, that is, patients doing poorly and dying on you. There are so many far-advanced brain tumors and so much major head trauma that you just accept it as an everyday occurrence. After the first few times, you don't get broken up by it. When you choose neurosurgery, you know that ahead of time. You don't get into this field if you can't handle that.

This is especially true at the Children's Hospital. I know it wipes some people out to work with these badly damaged kids or to watch a kid die. I've gotten to handle it by thinking of them as little adults. Even when I talk to the family, I tell myself these are the immediate relatives and not the parents of the kids. Otherwise, I might not be able to handle it. You can't just look at them as kids because they have maybe 60 years ahead of them that they have lost, and I tell myself that there are plenty of adults who come in and have very bad head trauma from a car accident that aren't going to make it, and that's a tragedy, too.

Some of this you pick up by watching the older attendings, but I think a lot of how you handle things is very individual and self-learned. That's why it's hard to be a good attending. They have to know where you are all the time in terms of your progress and let you do what you can to the limit of your abilities without intervening or interfering and then know when a resident is about to exceed his or her capabilities and step in without the resident's asking and before anything detrimental happens to the patient. A lousy attending is one who takes over and you're nothing but a scrub nurse. There's nothing that a resident hates more than preparing for a case, going over all the studies, reading up the night before, and then not being allowed to do a darn thing on their own in the operating room.

There's another kind of stress that attendings cause among the house officers that I doubt they're even aware of. Because all neurosurgeons are prima donnas, and because they have such big egos, they often get into differences about approaches and what is the best way to do something. If a resident gets to be associated with a particular attending or gets to be a favorite or operates with him a lot, the resident can get on somebody else's blacklist. It's like choosing sides between parents. This is bad and happens in a lot of programs. We have some of it here, but it's not nearly as bad as in some places.

You may not get the complete picture of the stress of training by just seeing the residents. Some of the residents are having a lot of second thoughts. They're faced either with quitting the field or heading for separation and divorce. There's tremendous stress in their marriages because of their work load and their fatigue. Most of us can handle the stress of the training. There are very few surprises. We knew what we were getting into. Where it becomes unbearable is when you're involved with a wife or a fiancée. Those women are under a lot of stress themselves and, in the process, create a lot of stress for the residents. The minimum amount you have to do in neurosurgery training would be insurmountable for most people, but we do it. However, you can't give your loved ones what they need and deserve. They have to get along a lot more on their own. Among the residents, even among those who are not thinking of quitting the field, many are thinking of divorce because of the tension.

I can honestly say that I'm not having any second thoughts even on one of those very bad on-call nights. I'm very pleased with my choice. A surgical specialty is what I wanted from the beginning. General surgery is work that is too gross. I like to do very fine things with my hands. Also, neurosurgery lends itself much more to an academic career, which is where I'm headed. That's one of the reasons I wanted this residency, because there is a heavy emphasis on research.

I do enjoy patient care very much and would never want to give that up completely, but what turns me on more than anything else is doing an original piece of work, carefully writing it up, and reporting it to my colleagues. That gives me a high. They have a neurosurgery residency where I went to med school. They can get you a job when you're finished with your training at half a million dollars a year. But nobody in the program ever goes into academics.

I can't explain it, but I get more gratification from presenting my findings to my colleagues and getting recognition from them than I get from
doing a good case in the OR.

▲   ▲   ▲

Let's pick up quickly on Dr. F.'s comment about neurosurgeons
being prima donnas and having big egos. Other house officers in this
specialty made the same observation, both about themselves and about
their teachers. Although this group of residents had more of a tendency
to express individual differences than in many specialties, they appeared
to be in consensus about the personality makeup of the typical neurosurgeon. For instance, Dr. V., a senior resident, had this to say about
neurosurgeons:

▼   ▼   ▼

That's not to say that all neurosurgeons are the same. Far from it.
They're extremely individualistic, and unlike in some specialties, it isn't simply a breakdown along full-time academics versus the private practice guys.
There is some of that. The private practice people are less uptight and more
fun. They say if there's a problem, we'll handle it one step at a time, and
there's less blaming and finger pointing. I guess the full-time people have to
look out for themselves in a political system.

But it's not black or white. There are some full-time people who are fun,
and there are some private guys that I will avoid at all costs because they're so
difficult to work with; one of my buddies did a beautiful piece of research for
which he won a national science award, but because he did it under the
'wrong' professor in the 'wrong' hospital here, he's had almost no local
recognition or reward. The University Hospital people are acting like it
doesn't exist. There's some long-standing conflict between many of the
leaders here, and no one knows why. Maybe they don't even remember
themselves anymore. Maybe it's just turf. Neurosurgeons are impossible,
and academic neurosurgeons are the worst. They have incredibly big egos,
and no department has enough space in it for them. They can clash over
anything. It's really silly because neurosurgery is like all medical specialties.
There are very few absolutes. There are very few clear-cut cures for any
disease. Yet, people take a hard-and-fast stand on something as being the
way, and they don't have a lot to back it up except their power and authority
and position.

▲   ▲   ▲

This view of neurosurgeons as being arbitrary, idiosyncratic, and highly territorial was viewed by most young house officers as also being ironic, as they had learned that much of what neurosurgeons are able to do is not as much curative as it is supportive in nature. Often, even supportive efforts are unsuccessful, considering the relatively high percentage of unsuccessful cures and lost patients. The house officers described this paradox as something they had discovered rather early in their training.

Dr. V. painted the picture this way:

▼　　　▼　　　▼

Your definition of success in neurosurgery changes as you go along through the years of training. At first, you have this Ben Casey image of all these miracle procedures. After a while, you get more conservative and are willing to settle for more modest outcomes. Certainly, with most of these malignant tumors of the brain, what you are doing is buying time for these people, and on the severe closed-head injuries, you can take care of the acute situation, but they have a long-term rehab experience ahead of them with very uncertain results.

I guess this is true in any specialty. If you start with some kind of white-knight expectation, you're headed for trouble. We have very few real cures in medicine. Mostly, you just stabilize people and keep them functioning if you can. That is most of medicine. In neurosurgery, maybe it's more obvious. You have to learn to say, 'This person has a very bad disease, and we can do something to make it a little less bad.'

The cases you really feel terrible about are the ones you tried so hard on and, despite that—well, maybe you missed a thing or two; most of these are aneurysms or arteriovenous malformations. You think you got them to the OR in time, and you think you got it all, but it turns out you really didn't, and at two o'clock in the morning, they bleed to death right in front of your eyes.

▲　　　▲　　　▲

The allusion to Ben Casey appeared more than once in these interviews. Dr. S., a second-year resident, had this to say on the subject: "It's funny, but when you try to recall your successes, nothing very dramatic sticks out. What I'm learning is that a lot of things we do are just palliative. Sure, we fix some backs and some necks, but most of what we do in the head is just temporary. We may add some time to somebody's life, but we don't cure too many brain tumor patients, and the more serious head injuries go on to lead very limited or impaired lives. A lot of the training leads you to look more realistically at what can be done and what the limitations are. You get the Ben Casey aura knocked out of you fairly early in the game. You learn to take care of extremely sick people, and you learn to accept death."

This cold inner realization of the limitations of neurosurgery, together with its daily frustrations and disappointments, did not prevent these young people from basking in the sunshine of the mystique enjoyed by their specialty. One young house officer said, "One thing I liked about neurosurgery was that it was a prestigious specialty. When you tell people you are in neurosurgery, their eyes light up, and they start to show more respect for you."

Along the same lines, another said, "Also, let's face it—there's a prestige aspect to neurosurgery. When you tell people you're in this field, they're a bit in awe of you. If you tell them you're in something like pediatrics, they say, 'Ho hum.' I must admit that was a factor, although I certainly wouldn't have chosen neurosurgery for that alone."

In daily practice, many experienced the work as a kind of emotional roller coaster with more lows than highs...but when the highs came, they were very high. Dr. V. said this:

▼   ▼   ▼

You've got to develop confidence in your own judgment gradually. That comes out of some experiences where you've proved yourself. I remember when I was on the VA rotation, there was this guy who we were sure was bleeding from somewhere. I felt certain from the clinical picture that it was an aneurysm, but we couldn't find it. People were ready to give up. I just kept insisting that we stay with it until we found it. It wasn't until the third angiogram that we were able to pinpoint it. Because of this, we were able to go in and get him clipped.

I have no doubt we saved this guy's life because there would have been a massive hemorrhage had we not done this. He ended up going back to his previous employment and is functioning as well as ever. That was a wonderful outcome. You don't need any drugs to get on a high after an experience like that.

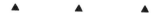

More often than not, the house officers were likely to find themselves in quite a different situation, one in which they were forced to proceed in the face of many imponderables and with the odds stacked against them. Dr. V. continued:

▼   ▼   ▼

Frequently, you find yourself in a scenario that goes something like this: It's 10 o'clock in the evening, and this patient comes in that you're pretty sure has an aneurysm that's leaking into his head. You have to decide what to do at 10 P.M. without being set up properly in the OR and having the right scrub nurses present who even know the names of all the instruments you'll be using, versus waiting until 7 A.M. when you are set up absolutely perfectly and have all the right people present and you know you can do a first-rate job. So, you sometimes put it off until morning and it turns out you shouldn't have.

But you also know if you had done it in the middle of the night, it might not have gone well anyway because you didn't have the A team. And you also know when you do these at two or three in the morning, you're less likely to spend the extra 10 or 15 minutes you might need to get something exactly perfect because you're so exhausted . . . and it may be those extra few minutes that will make the difference in the end, but you don't know it at the time. These things haunt you for a while afterwards.

▲   ▲   ▲

Dr. F.'s vivid description of his on-call experience with the CT scanner going down on him and many emergencies to be faced simultaneously is not an uncommon experience for these people.

Dr. S. added, "A neck injury can ruin your whole night and take all of your time and destroy any fantasy you had about a schedule for yourself. You can't leave that patient until everything is set. It may take three hours alone just to make the proper arrangements, just to get the right CT technician and get the scans done and the right radiologist to do the work for you, especially if it's late at night. Radiologists are basically lazy people, and it's hard to get them to come in for work when you feel you need them quickly. They usually try to talk you out of it. Then it takes time to deal with the anesthesia people, the OR nurses, and the families."

Dr. V. observed philosophically, "There's no doubt about the fact that this is a very stressful business, but we know pretty much what we're getting into ahead of time. There aren't too many surprises. I think our people deal with stress by staying inside themselves, remaining calm, and knowing what has to be done and then doing it."

The problem of dealing with the relatives of seriously impaired and perhaps permanently damaged patients was very stressful for these young people. This was true even if the patient was an adult, but if he or she was a child and the house officers had to deal with the parents, the stress was greatly magnified if the news was bad—and it often is. Again, Dr. S. had this to say about dealing with parents: "If it's a kid, it's much tougher. I do the best I can. Sometimes, the attending takes over, and I learn by listening to how they deal with parents. I can be off-the-cuff and straightforward with the families of adult patients, but with the kids, I have to rehearse every word I say before I walk in to see the family, and I'm still fairly uptight about it. My danger is that I tend to be overly optimistic and try to reassure the parents and then they expect too much. I paint too rosy a picture. One of the hardest things in the world is to tell parents that their kid isn't going to do well and may even die. I should learn better how to ease them into that slowly instead of clobbering them all at once at the end."

Dr. V. had other things to say about his work in pediatric neurosurgery, and these observations extended far beyond his less troubled work with parents and into his relationships with pediatric attendings, house staff, and nurses. In his own direct and unembellished fashion, he said:

▼   ▼   ▼

Some of the residents don't like to work with kids because they are too shaken by some of the outcomes and having to deal with the parents. I personally don't mind working with badly impaired kids or their families. I figure, as bad as things are, if it weren't for what I could do, they would be worse off, so I'm making things somewhat better for them. I can deal with that.

What drives me crazy at the Children's Hospital is the pediatricians and the nurses. I think people who go into pediatrics must be different from any other kind of doctor. They seem to be more patient advocates than physicians. The thing that's most distasteful about working at Children's is that you can't talk to the pediatricians straight. You can't say there is this kid with this kind of tumor in a certain place, and that such and such a procedure stands so much percentage chance of success, particularly if you add so many rads of radiation and such and such a course of chemotherapy. They act like you're some kind of monster if you talk like that.

But, if you say, 'Oh this poor little kid—what a tragedy. This poor dear child. We're going to do everything we can to save him,' and go on like that, then they think you're a good doctor. The nurses are even worse, and the ICU nurses are the worst of all. They swarm over these little kids in a way that is much worse than the families. They try to protect the kids from the doctors. It's like if you want to do some important procedure on them, you're the enemy and they have to defend the kids against you. I'd like to get rid of all the pediatricians at the Children's Hospital and fire the nurses and hire new ones. Then I think it would be a better place to work in. You shouldn't see behavior like this from professionals who have been working with very sick children for years.

I'm really comfortable with the kids and the parents. I'm honest with them and straight, and they understand me and we get along fine. With parents, there is almost no case where you can't give them some positive feedback and tell them something good about what's going on and what the chances are.

You can understand it when a parent gets very upset and very irrational and starts to scream at you. You can make allowance for that—I got kind of crazy when my *cat* got sick.

But professionals should know what the score is and act in a professional way. When I've mentioned this to some people down there, I just got blank stares. They don't seem to know what I'm talking about. It's like they don't fully appreciate what they can do and what they are there for. God, I remember this 13-year-old kid who was sent in from another hospital. He had had problems with coordination and headaches and nausea for three months. His school performance had gone way down. They had diagnosed him as meningitis. He had been brought in by helicopter as an acute emergency. When we scanned him in the ER, we could see that he had a tumor of the brain stem that was slipping into his spinal canal under great pressure. We took him directly to the OR, and we got him through all of that and he ended up going back to school and functioning very well. He's now three years postop and having no trouble. That's what this business is all about—and I didn't have to say [in falsetto], 'Oh, that poor child!'

▲   ▲   ▲

This criticism of pediatric staff is expressed by many in the surgical specialties. They see pediatric people as rather mushy-headed and acting sometimes as if no one else cared about the welfare of the kids but themselves. Surgeons find this offensive and not in the best interests of the child and the family.

Perhaps, there is a tendency for staff members engaged in the daily care of sick young children to become rather protective of them and to begin to experience a need to protect them from procedures perceived as unnecessarily invasive or painful.

Finally, there is the matter of marital and family life for these house officers. It was clear that, for many, spousal relationships were placed in serious jeopardy because of the incredible physical and psychological demands of this training. In many instances, marriages decompensated because neither partner was fully prepared for what would ensue once the house officer was deeply involved in training. It is only an impression, and to the best of my knowledge there are no formal studies on the subject, but it would appear that the marriages of these young people would stand a better chance of survival during training if childbearing is delayed and if the spouse has serious career commitments that consume time and energy and are in themselves a source of significant reward.

Chapter 10

OTOLARYNGOLOGY

Dr. Q. is a 29-year-old second-year resident in otolaryngology. He is divorced and has no children. The divorce occurred when he was in medical school. He has no family living in this area. He is of average build and dresses very neatly in color-coordinated shirt, tie, and slacks. His black hair is parted precisely in the midline. He wears wire-rimmed granny specs and is afflicted with the kind of beard that looks like five o'clock shadow at 9 A.M. regardless of how closely he shaves. Under this dark mask, his skin is like pale parchment. He spoke so quietly that I had to ask him to repeat his comments three or four times.

▼   ▼   ▼

I want to explain right off, if I sound kind of spacy, that I was on all day yesterday and today and on call last night with only about two hours sleep. On this service, when you're on call, you've got to cover not only the Eye-and-Ear Hospital emergency-room but also any ENT calls from the ERs at the University Hospital and Children's, too, plus any in-house consults that can't wait until morning, especially acute problems on the head and neck floor. You can even get called for severe nosebleeds on patients with bad clotting, as if this is an ENT problem, when, in fact, it is mostly a medical situation.

Because you're covering three hospitals, you're lucky to get four hours sleep. Usually it's much less. Last night, I had 8 or 10 emergency calls for such things as bad sore throats, ear infections, or nosebleeds that wouldn't stop.

You can also get called, especially at Children's, for a kid who is having trouble breathing and they are suspecting a foreign body in the pharynx or further down. I got called to Children's also for a kid on chemotherapy for leukemia who was draining pus from both ears and had a very bad white count. I had to suction out both ears and get him admitted before I finished with him. A little while later, I was called to Eye and Ear for a patient who had a laryngectomy a couple of weeks ago and whose tracheotomy tube had fallen out. Then there were two late admissions for surgery the following morning, and I had to work them up. Then back to Children's for a kid they thought had an epiglossitis. We couldn't get a decent airway into him, so I had to do a trache on him and admit him to the ICU for observation. I was up and down all night. The longest stretch of sleep was from 5 to 6:30—then I was up for good.

I suppose this sounds a little hairy, but I've learned that I work pretty well under stress even without sleep. I've learned that if I get into a bad situation, the adrenalin starts pumping. After it's over, you slow down and can't think as fast. It takes longer to make decisions, but I don't think I'm impaired. I think I still make the right decisions. I just need longer to do it. Maybe the most serious thing is that that affects your tolerance of people. I'm more irritable and can take less foolishness from the nurses, the interns, or patients with minor complaints who really don't need your time and are just doing a lot of whining and complaining. I get more quiet—less smiling and less talkative. I just hold back and try to suppress my irritation.

You don't think of ENT as having potential disasters, but we have carotid arteries blow on us all the time. Recently, on two on-call nights, I had the same lady blow her carotid artery on me twice, and I had to maintain pressure on it at 3 A.M. while we got the vascular surgeons in, got the attendings in house, got the OR rolling, got plastic surgery there, got her hydrated and central lines going, got hold of the anesthesia people, and so on. It can also be very scary when a kid has a bad anesthetic reaction after a simple T and A and almost dies on you. I haven't had a kid die, but I know other residents who have, and dealing with the family is quite an experience. Also, we see a lot of big-time airway problems because of aspiration of foreign bodies or because of anaphylactic problems.

I feel I'm in one of the top five programs in the country. It's very competitive getting into a residency like this. I'm proud to be a house officer in this department. Actually, it's getting more and more competitive all the time. When I applied, there were 430 applications for the 230 slots nationally. Now there are 1,000 for the same number. In fact, this is happening in all the surgical specialties. Who wants to be a general surgeon anymore? What you see is people bucking the national trend. There is pressure to expand the number of primary-care physicians, and what you have is a bunch of young people who want to be superspecialists.

The other thing that's driving people away from general surgery is the attitude in young doctors that medicine is a business. You want to get in there and make a good living and go home and see your family. A lot of the regulation that's being put on medicine is pushing people this way.

In fact, the real world is sort of scary out there, and there is not enough training of the residents to function in it with any business sense. That should be a part of every residency now. You have to face reality. A couple of

OTOLARYNGOLOGY

program chiefs have commented at national meetings that we are throwing our young, well-trained people out to the wolves. They are getting chewed up. Somebody totally ignorant of medicine, like somebody running a chain of proprietary hospitals, is going to dictate to you how to practice after you've spent 9 or 10 years learning how to do it. Like they're saying you have to send your tonsil and adenoid patients home because most of them do OK. But we know that the ones who do bad do real bad.

I'm sort of rattling on like this assuming you know the details of our training, which is probably not the case. Let's see if I can give you a quick overview. Training is broken into four-month blocks. I had my first four months on the head-and-neck cancer service as the junior house officer, then four months at Children's and four in the emergency room seeing everything that walks in the door—mostly routine and nonchallenging stuff. But it does give you a chance to catch up on your reading and your sleep.

Then, in your second year, you spend blocks at the VA, in the otology clinic, and back at Children's (but this four months is on maxillofacial plastic surgery), and a block of research time, and a chance to be chief resident rotating at Children's, University Hospital, and Eye and Ear, either as first assistant on very major cases or as the operator on less serious cases, and that depends entirely on the attending's judgment.

Three mornings a week you're in the OR. In the afternoons, you're working in one of the specialty clinics and working up patients for the next day's surgery. There are still a surprising number of tonsilectomies, adenoidectomies, and tympanectomies to do. Just by myself, I've done maybe 50 adenoidectomies and 75 tonsillectomies this year.

The clinics give you a broad exposure to different diseases. A lot of the clinic patients are much more complicated than the private patients because they tend to wait much longer to come for help, and things are more serious at that point, like tumors of the middle ear that may have been causing problems for a while. A private patient will get help quickly, but a clinic patient may wait so long that there is spread up toward the brain or into the inner ear, where surgery becomes a lot more delicate and tricky. That little area is a land mine. The whole space is only about 25 cubic centimeters. Anything interfering with it can give you big-time trouble. Right outside of it is the brain, the carotid artery, and sigmoid sinus, and the facial nerve, and you've got the auditory and vestibular systems involved. The number of things or combinations of things that can go wrong is almost endless.

This year, on Wednesdays, we get to be mostly observers in the OR on the most delicate kinds of surgery. We might be second or third assistant. We don't get to do much, but we watch techniques. I'm talking about vestibular nerve resections, cochlear implants, acoustic neuroma resections—major-league otology, not for junior residents to be playing around with. It's a little frustrating because you get to watch these things 7, 8, and 10 times without any hands-on involvement. There gets to be a limit on what you can learn just by watching, but there's no way a junior resident can be responsible for this kind of stuff. Your hands are just not ready to fool with this kind of stuff.

All these rotations at different hospitals and different clinics require adjustments on our part, but it's worth it. People don't realize how diverse ENT is. There are differences in what the private practitioners do, the head-and-neck cancer people, otology, the plastic specialists, the pediatric specialists, and so on. We get a very good flavoring, and I doubt you would get that if you stayed in one hospital. This was one of the reasons I wanted to come to this program. It has top people and the most diversity.

In spite of the fact that you work very hard, you are treated as a colleague by the faculty. We are invited to all the major conferences, and there is a lot of interest in our professional development.

Basically, I'm very pleased with the attendings. They're excellent technically and at transferring knowledge along with why something is done. They are patient with your questions and don't get annoyed. I'm the kind that asks a lot of questions. I also like somebody who can push you and make you think without harrassing you. We are very fortunate because most of the faculty measure up to these criteria. One of the attendings will come and sneak you away from the fellow who is doing a tonsillectomy and let you do a special case with him. He will help you through most of it and tell you what to say to the chief so that your butt is covered, and he seems to have done the case but actually you have done most of it under his supervision. That's a good attending. You would do any amount of scut work for that guy.

Once a year, you do get to sit down with the chief, and he goes over your evaluations from all the rotations. I did it recently, and we talked about everything but my evaluations, so I knew I was doing pretty good. Most of the feedback comes on rounds or in the OR. If you are doing anything out of line, they don't hesitate to let you know about it.

I've always known I wanted to be a surgeon. It was just a question of what kind. General surgery seemed too gross. I wanted to do finer work with all ages, from babies to geriatric work, and work that would allow some private time to set up a family, which general surgery or neurosurgery or cardiothoracic don't do. ENT just seemed the ideal choice for me.

I guess the major stress was one I didn't expect. The latest basic text in ENT contains 1,500 pages, and that is just the general text without all the subspecialties—plus all the journals that come out every month. It's pretty overwhelming.

They give us yearly examinations, and you have to score better than 50% of all the residents in the country or you are on probation. The chief reads off the scores with your name, and last year, he literally read out loud somebody's probation letter, so there's a lot of pressure on you.

The other pressure is just plain time. You have to staff all these services, and there are just not enough hours in the day. Somebody has to do the garbage work on the head-and-neck service. Somebody has to be in the ER to see all the routine stuff that comes in. It just has to be done. You are tempted to ask for extra people, but that's a two-edged sword. If you have a lot more residents, then you do fewer cases in the OR, and that's bad. Time in the OR is the bottom line, especially with hard cases. Also, you don't want to produce too many people. Then we would be like the general surgeons—in oversupply—and there won't be enough for us to do. Then you start super-specializing just to make a living, and that's bad for practice.

It's bad because there is already enough confusion in the minds of other physicians about how to use us, while, at the same time, we are developing esoteric fellowships like 'base of the skull' or 'microvascular surgery' fellowships. Yet, some things often get turned over to us that are so simple you can't believe it, like nosebleeds that anyone ought to be able to treat, or minor sore throats, or ear infections.

On the other hand, frequently we're not called when we ought to be. The general surgeons will try to change a trache tube on a new case where the incision hasn't healed sufficiently and they can't get the tube back in and the patient dies. That happened last week. GPs will see ear problems and give antibiotics and ear drops. Well, you don't give both. You give either one or the other, depending on where the problem is. One is for the outer ear, and one is for the middle ear. It just shows ignorance. Lots of pediatric residents will fumble around trying to get a foreign body out of a kid's ear and call us after three or four tries. By that time, the kid is off the wall and won't let you near him. So we end up having to take him to the OR and put him under general anesthesia. But you've got a kid who'll never let you near his ears again.

It is crazy, crazy. We are either underutilized or overutilized. I'm just amazed at how little most of the medical profession understands about this specialty.

▲   ▲   ▲

Dr. Q. presented us with such a detailed and factual description of the format of his training that it does not seem to require much amplification. His judgment that he was in one of the top programs in the country gave him a sense of pride and accomplishment. He acknowledged without remorse that his profession may be intentionally keeping down the number of trainees in order to prevent excessive competition, and he was willing to work much harder in the face of heavy demands because he, too, had an investment in seeing the field undersupplied with practitioners.

Like all of his brothers and sisters in the surgical specialties, he subscribed to the "bones-for-scut" philosophy. He was willing to perform all sorts of menial tasks that were below his level of training in order to be handed the scalpel in the OR and to be designated the primary surgeon on a case.

Dr. H., who was a fellow trainee in the program, stated that he was more than willing to accept the "bargain." As he put it, "You have to have the attitude that you are willing to do the scut work and that you will get the rewards for it in doing cases and getting teaching. Otherwise, you can get pretty unhappy, and I think this program is as good as any in keeping the bargain."

Dr. H. gave a wry description of how he learned whether or not he would be the primary surgeon on a case: "It is all tradition. When you walk into the OR how an attending positions himself around the table lets you know what you are going to do. Usually nothing is spoken. You may be the primary surgeon or not but you don't know until you are there, so you must be fully prepared to do anything. He may turn around and hand you the scalpel. When they think you are ready, they hand it to you. There's no discussion either before or after. I guess it's not a bad idea. It keeps you on your toes. You have to do your homework."

Dr. H.'s best remembered case was actually one in which he should have been better prepared but wasn't. On his new assignment as chief resident on the head-and-neck service and on his first day in the operating room, he found himself in the OR with a senior attending and was told to do a neck dissection on a very difficult and complex cancer case. He went on, "Having been off the service for a long time, you just don't see cases like that. That was really a curve ball. I wasn't as prepared as I should have been because I didn't expect to be doing it, so I sort of stumbled through it. But in the end, it went fine. It just took twice as long as it should have. Looking back, maybe it wasn't all that difficult a case, but it was both challenging and fulfilling to me because I didn't fall on my face and I was able to handle it. It isn't too hard to lose control of a major vessel in a situation like that, and then you may have major bleeding on your hands. And you have a similar risk with the nerve supply. It's easy to section a major nerve without knowing it if you don't know your way around. Then you really have a disaster on your hands."

As I listened to these surgical trainees, regardless of their particular specialty, I sensed over and over how much they enjoyed stretching themselves, walking on the edge of their knowledge and ability, taking calculated risks—and, in the end, landing on their feet.

The kinds of patients who seemed much less rewarding to them were those with more ambiguous types of disorders that were hard to nail down and hard to arrive at firm decisions about with respect to surgery. Dr. H. described these very well as follows: "The two kinds of patients that give me a headache are, first, the patients who complain of dizziness when you can't find any physical abnormalities. How do you tell a patient he is not dizzy when he says he is but you can't find anything wrong? So your treatments get to be pretty empirical. Sometimes you help, but sometimes you don't. The other type is the terminal cancer patient with chronic pain, which is so hard to evaluate. Patients have such different thresholds of pain. I know they have cancer, but some have little or no reason for so much pain following surgery, even after several weeks. There is no organic reason for the number of complaints that you hear, and it is extremely difficult to evaluate them. Some are really not terminal at all, and you don't want to get them addicted to drugs."

With few exceptions, work with infants and children proved to be a major component of practice in otolaryngology. Attitudes about this work varied considerably. Dr. Q. appeared to have more difficulty with his pediatric counterparts than with the children themselves. Dr. H. had apparently decided that, although he enjoyed children, he would not want to do much work in pediatric ENT because, "One of the hard things is dealing with the parents, who are sometimes so uptight and anxious that they get irrational and they ask you questions to which there aren't any answers. Or they ask you irrelevant questions, and you have to figure out where they are coming from. Or they get very picky and demanding and start focusing in on some tiny little thing that doesn't matter and they lose sight of the bigger picture."

Once more, what seems obvious to the casual observer is that these surgical house officers had received no training in dealing with anxious or demanding parents and relatives. They seemed unwilling or unable to look beyond the overt questions, to help the individual ask what might really be bothering her or him and to attempt to respond satisfactorily.

In fact, the less sophisticated and less educated patients may have been valued more because the house officers had more responsibility for them if they were in lower socioeconomic groups and because, as Dr. Q. stated, clinic patients tended to present with more complex and serious disorders and might be better teaching cases for that reason.

The house officers did not complain about inadequate supervision in the management of difficult families. They were more likely to complain about the absence of training in the business aspects of practice management because they saw the field as one in which economic survival was becoming more stressful every year.

They asked for seminars or courses in financial planning, in staff recruitment and personnel practices, and in marketing. Dr. Q. described some recent graduates as "getting chewed up" out there. He decried the fact that individuals operating large hospitals as invester-owned corporations are in a position to dictate some aspects of medical practice about which they know almost nothing.

Although many of the house officers in otolaryngology were planning to pursue subspecialization through fellowship training after their residency, some were simultaneously upset about the fact that their work had become so narrow and focused that outsiders, even other physicians, knew very little about what they were doing. As Dr. Q. concluded, this ignorance led to abuse and misuse of his potential contribution to patients. He often ended up feeling that he had been called to help in cases where others should have known what to do, and that his contribution had not really utilized the skills of someone in his specialty. At the same time, his frequent experience was that he was called so late that he might be faced with trying to undo a potential medical disaster. He was troubled, as were many specialists and subspecialists, that his colleagues in other disciplines did not know how to use him very well or very efficiently.

Chapter 11

OPHTHALMOLOGY

Dr. B. is a 38-year-old first-year resident in ophthalmology. He had originally been trained as an optometrist, a profession he had practiced for several years before going to medical school. He is obviously older than most of his peers. There is a calm, settled quality about him. He is sandy-haired with a light sprinkling of gray at the temples, and he wears rimless glasses. He is rather soft-spoken, which was a bit of a problem because our interview took place in the evening in the emergency room of the Eye and Ear Hospital. Intermittently, the PA system blared in the background, nurses shouted to each other up and down the hall outside the office, children cried or screamed in the waiting room, and there were constant phone interruptions. Dr. B. dealt with all of this with equanimity.

▼　　　▼　　　▼

This whole specialty is undergoing an evolution. I'm working in a hospital, but I almost never have a patient who has been admitted to the hospital. The whole specialty is becoming ambulatory. You are either dealing with emergency-room or clinic patients, or you're doing outpatient surgery. Even the trauma cases like auto accidents tend to have multiple traumas involving plastic surgery, fractures of facial bones, skull fractures, and so on. Therefore, we are only ancillary consultants if there is some eye damage. As it works out, they are almost always admitted to somebody else's service. Partly, this is what cost containment has done, but it's also due to advances in laser surgery.

What has happened is that you can no longer bring people into the hospital because of their eyes. They are just not sick enough. And anybody who is is probably eligible for somebody else's service, not yours. Once in a while, we admit somebody to the hospital if they have a very severe corneal ulcer or blood in the interior chamber of the eye.

During my year of training, I've seen about 35 to 45 patients a day in the ER. A good 60% of them suffer from external eye disease. The others complain of ocular pain of unknown origin where they have retinal disease or cataracts. You also have to do any in-hospital consultations at the University Hospital, and if there are any admissions to Eye and Ear, you have to help with the histories and physicals on the private patients.

As I said, most of your time is spent seeing patients either in the general eye clinic or in specialty clinics like the retinal clinic or the plastics clinic.

I'm aware that a lot of what I'm doing, I have really done before in one way or another. I was working in a hospital in Colorado where I had lots of contact with medical students and junior ophthalmology residents, and I realized I knew as much as or more than they did about a lot of things, and yet I couldn't do many of the things they were doing, like assisting in surgery. I decided when I was almost 30 that it was time to take the plunge and go to medical school. I was turned down the first two years and finally made it on the third try. I don't have any regrets about it now, although sometimes these days I get a little bored and I feel like I'm not challenged enough. Lots of times you are working in the ER and you're seeing all the walk-ins, stuff that could be done by a nurse: foreign bodies in the eye, minor infections, that kind of stuff. Maybe only about 5% of what I see I haven't seen before, and I'll bet that only about 60% or 70% of what walks in needs to be seen by a physician anyway.

Maybe that statement was a little extreme. In some ways, I'm not as bored as I may seem. I have to remember that I spent four years in medical school and one year in a general surgery internship, and that there has been something of a revolution in ophthalmology in those five years. There have been so many advances in technology, so many things I never heard of or didn't know about that I really do have a lot of new stuff to learn, stuff I was never exposed to before. There are lots of new drugs that didn't exist previously and lots of new instruments and techniques.

That business of having to see everything that walks in the door is kind of a sore point with the first-year residents. There is no reason we couldn't have a nurse screen out a lot of that simple stuff. Most of us feel that we can't learn anything from it, and it's a waste of time in our learning process. Sure, to get a sense of total eye care, you need to see a little bit of everything once, but whether you need to see a lot of everything a lot of times is a real question.

My last assignment was in pediatric ophthalmology. It was an interesting experience because you have to learn how to manage those kids to examine them and to do procedures. I learned an old adage in ophthalmology that says, 'One toy, one look.' So, you come in with a bag of toys, and for each toy you let them play with, you can get a quick look at the eye. If you've got a bag of toys, you can get a bag of looks with most kids. Also, if you learn to make a certain number of strange noises and act a little crazy, that is also distracting and helps you sneak quick looks at both the external and the internal eye, and it doesn't take very long, if you get experienced, to see what you want to. I ended up liking it very much, and I may be headed for a fellowship in pediatric ophthalmology. It's tougher to work with the parents because you have to follow through, and to get a three-year-old to wear glasses is something you just dump in the parents' lap and they have to handle it. Sometimes, you can get a dose from them.

Being on call can be a strange experience. I think the temperature has a lot to do with being on call, since it is almost all emergency room. If the temperature is over 70 degrees and it's dry outside, you end up with 20 or 30 people to see, most of them before one o'clock in the morning, but a few during the night. If it's raining and 50 degrees, like it is right now, it will be a slow night. Lots of people finish work at odd hours and drift past the hospital and see the sign and think to themselves this is a good time to get their eyes looked at because they have been irritated or sore and they can't see well. Lots of intoxicated people come in with foreign bodies in their eyes. If the weather is not so good, you just don't see very many of these people.

There is no doubt about the fact that there is a lot of reward and instant gratification in ophthalmology. That's probably why people go into it. It's a finite field. You can learn most of what you need to learn pretty quickly, and you can see results. A lot of people are sort of wired up that way and need that kind of professional life.

We really get thrown into it in the first year of training. We don't have much one-on-one with attendings because it's all ambulatory stuff and emergency room. I'm kind of impressed that some first-year residents who haven't had the experience I've had can get thrown in here cold and manage somehow, because I myself sit here some nights looking at something and wondering what's going on and not being able to figure it out; even to describe what is going on, what you are looking at, so you can talk to the attending on the phone sometimes is confusing.

It's a whole new vocabulary, and in med school you may spend only two or three weeks on that service and have forgotten most of it anyway. Ophthalmology is a very restricted field. It doesn't go out of its way to educate a lot of people or to interface with other specialties. In some ways, it's pretty isolated from the mainstream of medicine. But the checks and balances here are pretty good, and people can't get too far off target without being checked or corrected. A large part of it is knowing when to ask for help, and I guess that is what you learn more in the first year than anything else.

There is enormous variation in the attendings, even though the group is not very large. Some you can call up and talk to on the phone one-to-one like a colleague. Even if you are a first-year resident and you are struggling and you don't even know exactly what to call things, they will sort of help you along with it. Others just seem to make you feel stupid, like you should know all of this from the beginning and it's your fault if you don't. For them, there is a kind of hazing quality to this. Word gets around pretty quickly among the residents about who's who among the attendings. But I think this program is better than many. There is kind of a low-key quality to it without too many Type A people. You know the ones who say, '*I* did it; now *you're* going to suffer.'

All in all, I think this is kind of a low-stress training program and a low-stress specialty. For instance, I don't think there is any real drug or alcohol abuse in this department. I might not know it if it was going on, but I think I would notice if somebody came in functionally impaired in the morning, and I never see that. Personally, I am very careful. I might have two or three beers during a whole week, but I will never even have one drink before I'm to be on. I think most of us are very conscientious about that. This may not be true in some other departments that I've heard about, but I would be very surprised if anything was going on here.

I had some experience with drugs a long time ago as a kid in college, and I don't know how you could pull off this kind of work and get away with it if you were on anything. I just don't think it's possible. I'm on call every sixth night and every sixth weekend. Maybe that doesn't sound like much, but it is because you lose sleep, and it takes a few days to catch up at my age. How could any of us be fooling around and get away with it? You've got to be as sharp as you can. You owe it to yourself, and you owe it to the people you see.

I guess the major stress for me is that I feel out of synch. The content of the residency itself is not so bad. It's that I'm too far advanced. It's very difficult for me. Some days it really gnaws at me. I keep thinking about if I could only do it all over again.

I'm sort of champing at the bit to get to those final years of training when I will be doing lots of eye surgery of different types. This is what I wanted to do in the first place when I went to medical school. All this is leading up to it. I guess I've got to pay my dues and put my time in so I can do the heavy stuff later.

Even then, I will still have a way to go. I'm planning a postresidency fellowship, probably in pediatric ophthalmology. I look around me at my contemporaries, who are now in their late 30s, are settled in their practice, and are financially well off, and I haven't even started yet. I will be past 40 when I finish training. Every once in a while, I do have some doubts about what I'm doing.

Sometimes I think, 'Why me? Why couldn't I get my head together when I was 18 or 19 and start off on the right track?' Maybe I'm just the kind of guy who has to arrive at a goal through a roundabout course. If I had gone straight through, I would have missed a lot of the experiences both professionally and personally that I have had, the chance to travel, to work in other settings, to meet lots of different people. People who stay right on the pre-med and med-school track straight through still are being told where to go and what to do, and your life is very structured and you have comparatively little autonomy. It's kind of a prolonged adolescence. That's what I'm experiencing now as I've gone back into training.

You feel a little schizophrenic. You go home and you are a father and a husband and a homeowner and a taxpayer and so on, and you come to work and some attendings treat you like you are a 14-year-old kid.

▲   ▲   ▲

Although Dr. B. was not a typical resident in many regards, I chose his interview to reproduce *in toto* because he was articulate in describing the ups and downs of training and, for me, placed it in a rather clear perspective.

To the rank outsider, it may come as something of a shock to learn that ophthalmology, a specialty that concerns itself with roughly one cubic inch of the body, now has generated eight subspecialties. Some residents described how little contact they had with attendings in their first year of training because it was all so general and how much this contact increased as they moved into the subspecialty areas. I was not aware, for instance, that one could be a specialist in glaucoma or in external eye disease or in the cornea or in the retina or in neurological diseases associated with the eye. Nor was I aware that between one half and two thirds of the house officers go on to do fellowships in one of the subspecialty areas.

One house officer talked about how strange it felt not to do rounds every morning, as that had been a part of his life as a medical student and intern. This, of course, is the inevitable result of having no beds in the hospital and becoming strictly an ambulatory specialty. As short a time as three years ago, residents pointed out that there would be, on any given day, 20 or 30 patients in the hospital. Most felt that this was not a problem, that these patients were not really very sick, didn't have to come into the hospital, and didn't need acute care. Most felt that care was not compromised and that it was a good idea to stay out of the hospital if possible. One laughingly repeated the adage, "Hospitals are no places for sick people."

Most of this group of house officers was basically pleased with that training and with the department in which they served. In more than one instance, however, they were highly critical of the nonclinical people who staffed the front door of the hospital. One said in reference to this: "If I were the boss, I would fire all the people that had anything to do with greeting patients at the door, doing the paperwork, doing the financial interviewing, doing the reception, and so on. They are cold, bored, and uninterested and make everybody feel unwelcome. No matter how good the rest of the staff is, if that first person you meet when you walk in the door doesn't handle you right, you have a sour taste in your mouth. Nobody smiles. They look up at the patients as if they were interfering with their work."

The house officers did not view their superiors as particularly warm, friendly beings, although they were pleased with the training they were receiving. One house officer said, "You have to remember that ophthalmologists are microsurgeons. They have tighter sphincters than most people, including general surgeons. That's reflected in their personalities. They are more uptight and harder to deal with. For that reason, I don't know if I would want to go into academics. I don't know if I would want to get involved with the personalities of a department and the politics of medical school. When you're dealing with ophthalmologists, I'm not sure it's worth it."

All of the house officers in this group stated emphatically that they could not conceive of their colleagues abusing drugs or alcohol and being able to function on a daily basis. I suspect from the nature of the work I heard described that this is an accurate observation. Microsurgeons are microsurgeons!

Yet, these young people could not be stereotyped. Dr. B., who enjoyed so much working with children and who was planning a fellowship in pediatric ophthalmology, was very different from Dr. L., a 28-year-old second-year resident, who said, "I've seen lots of kids in the emergency room and some during my internship. I like kids but I don't like to examine them. It is extremely hard to examine a little kid's eyes. In the end, you have to put them in a papoose and put some anesthetic in their eyes and prop the lids open with an instrument before you can really look, and the whole time they are screaming and struggling and there really isn't much you can do about it. The procedure really feels very invasive to them. I don't see myself in pediatric ophthalmology. I just don't have the patience for that."

As the reader will discern, it is not only impossible to stereotype trainees within a given program, it is inappropriate to say that all surgical trainees are similar. For instance, the contrast between house officers in otolaryngology and ophthalmology and those in orthopedic surgery (see the next chapter) would probably be obvious to the average child of eight!

Chapter 12

ORTHOPEDIC SURGERY

Dr. U. is a tall, muscular young man with coal-black hair, gray-green eyes, and olive skin. He speaks with a slight accent, which I could not identify, and told me simply that he had grown up in a mining town in Pennsylvania and that his parents rarely spoke English in the home. He has outsized hands and feet. His movements are controlled and very economical. There doesn't appear to be any wasted motion. On his wrist was a watch that would look enormous on mine. It bristled with buttons and an electronic calculator. A bush of dark hair stuck out from above the V neck of his scrub shirt. When he crossed his legs, I saw 12 inches of sockless calf ending in scruffy docksiders.

▼   ▼   ▼

I'm 30 years old, and I'm in my fifth year. I'm now a chief resident. The program consists of two years in general surgery first and then three years of orthopedics.

Actually, the first two years in general surgery were harder. You are into more life-threatening situations. Many more things can go wrong that are catastrophes, and also, you are younger and less experienced yourself. The last three years are not nearly as tough. It's pretty hard to kill an orthopedic patient unless you are awfully stupid.

Although there is a lot of orthopedic knowledge, most people who are not in this specialty don't have any idea of that. We seem to have the image of not having to know very much, but that isn't true. I guess it used to be that the guys who went into orthopedics were the bottom 10% of the class and strong as an ox.

We cover eight hospitals, so we have enormous patient volume. In several of these hospitals, the emergency rooms are very busy. I like covering eight hospitals because we get to do stuff in earlier years that you would have to wait until your last year to do, like doing a total joint.

As a chief resident, you have lots of responsibility for teaching junior residents. You have to make sure the OR runs smoothly. In some hospitals, you have your own clinic, and you are the only guy there, although you can call an attending on the phone if you want to. I get to do lots of surgical procedures on those patients with an attending assisting.

The residents think that we cover eight hospitals in the city because the chief wants only one training program. So we brought all of them into our orbit. The advantage is not only more time in the OR, but also each has its own different attendings who specialize in different areas. One hospital is strong on total joint replacement. Another is big on arthritis. Another one is very big on trauma cases. I guess the big disadvantage is that you are constantly getting used to new people and new administrative procedures and different medical records and so on.

The attendings in these hospitals vary a lot. You can learn as much by watching somebody who is making mistakes as by watching somebody who is very good if you know what you are looking at. The more senior you are as a resident, the more you become aware of the mistakes that attendings make. You try not to repeat them.

At the hospital I am assigned to now, there is enormous volume and few residents. You start rounding at 6 A.M., and there is a conference at 7 A.M., and then you have to be in the OR all day after that, often till 6 P.M. So the typical day varies tremendously, depending on where you are. After the OR, you have to work up new patients for the next day's surgery. The number of admissions can vary from maybe 4 to 13 or 14. To tackle that after a full day's surgery is really a head knocker.

On Sunday, when you are on alone, you have to work up all the new admissions for the next day, not just the one's of your attending. That could be as many as 22 in some places. All you can do is check them out—listen to their hearts and lungs, examine them for what they came in for, and take a brief history. If you pick up anything, you have to get a consult quickly, but there's not too much of that. That's the other thing about orthopedic patients: they are mostly healthy people medically, so you don't run into a lot of complications.

I went into this specialty because I like working with my hands and could probably have been happy in any surgical specialty, although general surgery is pretty hopeless these days in terms of the job market. Orthopedics is more interesting than people think. There are lots of new procedures coming along every day, like total replacement of joints or arthroscopy, and you get to take care of patients of all ages, from very old people to kids. I especially enjoy working with kids, and there is a lot of that in this business because there are so many babies born with congenital deformities that you have to work with.

My work with kids is very satisfying. My rotation at the Children's Hospital was one of the most enjoyable ones. Also, Children's is one of the easier hospitals because you may have only 30 patients to round on there. At others, you may have as many as 60 or 70. When that happens, not an awful lot of teaching can go on because of the number of patients.

The rounding at Children's can be difficult for other reasons because, although the kids are often asleep when you round early in the morning or late in the evening, the parents are there and we get a lot of questions. Lots of them are lower-income families with low education, and the questions are unsophisticated or off-center and show a lot of fear. You think you have explained everything, and then they come out with a question that shows they don't understand. So you go back and explain again. Recently, we had to add a little wire to one kid's bone in order to strengthen it. We hadn't originally planned to do that. The parent asked me, 'Did this mean that the kid had cancer of the bone?' I was really taken aback.

Often the biggest job with children is nonoperative. It's taking care of closed fractures with lots of casting. Also, there is lots of work on club feet that involve casting. Sometimes you have to take a kid to the OR even if surgery isn't indicated because you can't work with the kid awake. You have to put him to sleep. There are also a fair number of clubfoot operations, back operations, and congenital hip abnormalities.

This is pretty hard physical work in orthopedics—I mean in the OR. You learn to deal with your own backaches and leg cramps. You just sort of ignore them after a while. You learn to work with a full bladder and an empty stomach because operating-room time is everything when you are in training. You just ignore the physical discomforts.

But as I said, it can be very satisfying. Recently, I was the primary surgeon on a kid where we had to realign the hip and cut off a good bit of bone. It changed the angles of how things fit together, so that the hip was more functional and the child could have normal activity. This involved a good bit of judgment about how to cut and at what angles, so things would fit perfectly. The attending let me do it, and I said this is what I want and this is how I want to do it, and he said go, and everything went perfectly. I think he would have done it differently, but he let me go my way. Afterward, the junior resident said that was perfect. How did I know what to do? He said that's how it should be done, smooth and fast. He doesn't know how much homework I did and how much thinking I did about it ahead of time.

Surgery can also be a humbling field. Every time things go well and you have a case like that one, something comes along that ought to be easy and turns out to be a terrible headache. You don't know why, but it keeps you honest. Just when you think everything is going well in replacing a total joint, you will crack the bone, and you have to try to put all the pieces together again to make it work.

To be honest, most people go into surgery because it is a bit of a high. You see a lot of people in pain and you can give them quick relief. You can fix things quickly and see immediate results. There's a lot of hands-on work, and you know you are fixing things. If it is a good result, people are grateful and happy.

This residency is loose. If you wanted to sneak through, you could. Nobody is on you to tell you when you have to read such and such. A lot of it, you are on your own. Twice a year, you meet with a department committee, which is supposed to review your progress, and they go over your evaluations from all the hospitals. But the most constructive criticism comes on rounds or in the OR. That's where the attendings can eyeball what you are doing.

And we can eyeball them, too. We know who is willing to put out for the residents and shares knowledge and experience without your having to pull teeth. I have a tendency to ask a lot of questions, and I can tell if the attending is getting annoyed with me. I've got to feel free to ask why are we doing it this way instead of that way and have him explain it to me even if I don't agree. I want the attending to take the time to share his or her thinking. Whether or not you get this from an attending varies a lot. In some of the smaller private hospitals, some of these people are just out to make money. They want to see the patients and go home. Maybe only about 15% or 20% of these people would I go to or send my kid to. That's really for a lot of different reasons, like some of them don't show up to see the patient after surgery. With some, it's their personality. They are just not nice people.

When I went into orthopedics, I wanted to be a complete doctor—you know, read the X rays, read the EKGs, treat their heart disease if they had it. Well, you just can't do that. There is no time. Now, we just routinely get a medical consult on anybody over 60 whether they need it or not. In effect, you are getting a medical house officer to work up the patient for you because you have to play it safe in that age group. What happens after a while is you get deskilled in these areas. If you don't do it enough, then you forget how to do it well.

When you get into any surgical specialty, you have to be prepared to work long hours. I get up at 5:15 every morning. You have to have a high energy level and be able to get along on not very much sleep. The work doesn't get much less as you get older. If you can't handle that, you shouldn't be in a surgical specialty.

Your life gets pretty stretched out. I'm married and I have a child, so what free time I have goes to my family. My wife was a lawyer who stopped working when our child was born. But she keeps me honest. I can't talk a lot of medical mumbo jumbo at home. I have to speak in simple language. It has helped me to talk to families and to patients. I do try to keep in shape by running or exercising. Some of the time, you just want to sit back and watch TV and become a vegetable.

I guess I'm one of the few in my group who are going out into private practice. Most of them are going into subspecialty training. I plan to join a private orthopedic group and do full-time practice. I like taking care of patients and seeing a lot of them. I don't want to spend my time doing research. Even the fellowships seem too narrow for me. There are fellowships on the spine, one on the hand, one on sports medicine, one on total joints, one on pediatrics. I don't want to restrict my professional life that way. I think I know something about all of those things, and I would like to do something in each area when I'm finished. I'm sure going to try.

▲   ▲   ▲

Because this is the last of our surgical specialties, it becomes easy to see how much these house officers have in common. Therefore, I will not tread once more well-worn pathways.

Nevertheless, there is always something fresh and different to learn from each of these specialties and from each group of house officers. What emerged for me from orthopedic surgery was that it seemed to attract young people who were very active physically, and who had at least some interest in sports medicine, in children, and in correcting physical disabilities. It is perhaps the most "mechanical" of the specialties, not in the sense that the practice itself is mechanical, but in the sense that it must be concerned with how the bony skeleton works, its joints and articulations, and how its various muscle groups function together to allow for proper body posture, movement, and control. Perhaps, if these people were not interested in medicine, they might well go into architecture or engineering as careers.

The general sense of being rather superior as people seemed pervasive in this group. At worst, it could be displayed as a kind of arrogance. At its best, I saw a self-image characterized by calm in the face of adversity; physical stamina in the face of demands that would defeat most people; a very high threshold to physical pain and discomfort; and a philosophical attitude about victory and defeat that permitted the house officer to move on to the next challenge without being crushed by the loss of a patient or the failure of an operation.

For instance, in response to my usual question about the use of drugs or alcohol in the peer group, Dr. E., a 33-year-old chief resident in orthopedic surgery, said, "I've never seen anything that makes me suspicious. I never see anybody drunk or impaired in any way. We do party a bit, but most of it is beer drinking on the weekends. Nobody shows up under the weather for work. The peer pressure in our department is such that people just couldn't do it. You would be looked down on as a kind of low character. You couldn't survive in our group. I know that I don't want to associate with people like that. We all feel that way."

Dr. E., in the same interview, when discussing his plans for future practice and the unattractiveness of routine orthopedics (in contrast to sports medicine, which he found very attractive), said, "Originally, I was interested in spinal surgery, but I don't like the population of people you meet there. In the end, you work with a lot of people who are trying to get out of doing what they are supposed to do, and there is lots of litigation. The paperwork is terrible, and you are in court and with lawyers. That isn't the way I want to spend my life. It's real tough to take care of a lot of these chronic low-back-pain patients. In sports medicine, you can usually do something. I don't like working with patients where I have to say that we don't know what's wrong, that we've tried everything and we don't know why there is still pain and there isn't anything to offer. We call them low-back losers. Hell, I have low back pain from all the sports I've played, but I can stand over the operating table and manipulate limbs all day, and you just sort of live with the pain. It's no big deal if you are doing something you want to do. It's hard to have sympathy for people who have some pain and sort of give up living. They seem to think that society has to support them just because they have some pain. I'm kind of hard-core when it comes to this. I don't think they should be drawing money from people who want to work or people who are really disabled and can't work. If you see 10 of those patients in a row, it really wears you out. They have their family there and their wives, and they bring their little kids in to play on your sympathy."

All of the orthopedic house officers I spoke with enjoyed their work with infants and children because they saw themselves as restoring these disabled kids to a normal or a near-normal life, one in which the physical activity and freedom of childhood would become more available to them.

To a person, they resented the stereotype that had apparently been held of individuals who chose orthopedic surgery in the past as physically strong but not terribly bright. In fact, many resented the stereotype of surgeons in general. One put it as follows: "I'm not sure it's true that surgeons like to make rapid decisions and act on them without thinking a great deal. I think really good surgeons plan ahead and think of all the options and decisions that may have to be made once they get into the operating room. They ask themselves, 'What will I do if this happens and what will I do if that happens?' so that when they are actually performing surgery, it looks like they are making rapid decisions, but they have thought it all out."

Although they complained a bit about feeling harassed because they had to cover eight hospitals in their training period, most saw advantages in being exposed to so many different attendings and in functioning in different settings that had different foci of activity. They did not seem to mind so much running from hospital to hospital because in one place they could learn a great deal about arthritis; in another, about trauma surgery; in a third, about joint replacement; and so on. Again, the world had become so subspecialized for these young people that they did not seem to be able to get anything they needed for their basic specialty training in one center.

Therefore, they constantly functioned under the pressure of sub-specializing too early in their training, knowing more and more about less and less while facing the day when they would have to enter practice and be able to handle any patient who walked in the door if they were to earn a living. The alternative was to seek an academic career in a medical center. Many did not feel temperamentally suited to this or did not see themselves as competitive in the research arena or in the political environment that characterizes academic life.

Part III

THE "HOSPITAL-BASED" SPECIALTIES

There is a group of specialties that the medical profession has labeled in shorthand the *hospital-based specialties*. These include anesthesiology, radiology, and clinical pathology. On the surface, they would appear to have little in common. They do share several important characteristics, however.

Perhaps their most typical feature is that, with few exceptions, most practitioners in these three specialties play supportive roles to their colleagues in the medical and surgical areas. That is, the usual pattern of practice is that they serve patients who are the primary concerns of other physicians.

As their label indicates, these specialties are hospital- or institution-based, although this is not universally the case. By the nature of their clinical practice, they require large amounts of highly technical equipment, trained allied health professionals, and complex data-storage systems.

Although their functions are critical to the conduct of modern medical practice, they tend to play out their daily roles to some degree in the background and without a front-line clinical role as the patient's physician of record.

Chapter 13

ANESTHESIOLOGY

Dr. R. is a 30-year-old, recently married senior resident in anesthesiology. He was dressed in the uniform of the day: blue scrub suit, white lab coat, stethoscope draped around his neck, pager clipped to the pocket of his coat, and well-worn Nikes. He is tall, slender, and Nordic-looking. Uncharacteristically, he appeared 10 minutes early for his interview, breezing into my outer office just as I was getting off the phone there. This took him by surprise, as he was eating an ice-cream popsicle (his lunch). He explained that he had expected to sit quietly for 10 minutes and enjoy his ice cream. Although I invited him to bring it into the office with him, he insisted on dumping it into the wastebasket so that it would not interfere with the interview. He is soft-spoken but articulates clearly and to the point. There was no evasiveness around sensitive issues and no effort to rush through the interview despite his hectic schedule.

▼   ▼   ▼

This residency is changing in a lot of ways. I'm in the last class where training will be for three years. Everybody after us will have four years. I really don't know the reason for this because I can't see what they're adding to the program that's very crucial; it seems to be mostly a bunch of electives. I suspect the actual reason is that they want to slow down the flood of anesthesiologists going into practice because there are too many now. This means that, for a whole year, at some point in the near future, no one will be graduating.

For me, this last year involves several months on pediatric anesthesiology, some time in critical-care medicine, and some experience in the pain clinic. My current assignment is cardiac and thoracic surgery. This mostly involves cardiac transplants, an occasional heart–lung transplant—we even did a Jarvik-7 implant yesterday; we've done several pulmonary lobectomies for people with lung cancer, and so on.

The most stressful times are during induction, when you are putting the patient under, and during emergence, when you are bringing the patient out. Once you have the patient fairly stable and at a good level for surgery, you are sort of monitoring the various functions and things go fairly well.

We're giving them various medications that depress their body functions; that means we have to take over those functions for them, especially respiration and circulation. So in effect, we're 'running' the patient's body while he or she is under this kind of surgery. You have to keep track of urine output, all the blood chemistries; in essence, you are keeping an eye on the physiology of the body and doing whatever manipulations are necessary, both mechanically and chemically, to keep the patient stable and out of trouble.

There's a saying in anesthesiology that the best preoperative medication is careful discussion with the patient the night before. You've got to deal with all their anxieties and questions so you can reduce the tension and get them loosened up. Then they need a lot less 'tranquilizing.' Also, you've got to spend a fair amount of time with them checking into smoking history, asthma, emphysema, urinary tract infections; and you have to spend time carefully looking at their airway so you can anticipate any problem with intubation. You look for false teeth and caps to make sure you don't break anything loose—and if you do, you can get it, and it doesn't show up in the patient's chest X ray after the surgery.

Maybe the surgeons ask a lot of the same questions, but they don't take the time to write them on the chart, so you don't have the information. Obese patients are very hard to manage because it's a lot harder to get into their airway, and they also have a lot more weight bearing down on their chest. The anesthesiologist's nightmare is putting a patient to sleep, having him stop breathing on you, and then not being able to get an airway in.

The toughest thing you have to do in the evenings is getting informed consent from the patients. It's walking a tightrope. You don't want to scare them to death about all the possible complications of surgery and anesthesia, but you do have to give them a basic understanding of the risks. Most patients take it pretty well and understand you're carrying out your medical and legal responsibilities. I walk them through it and try to find out whether they are irrational about things or whether they have accurately heard what I've told them, whether there are any fantasies remaining about all the horrible things that are going to happen to them. I try to give them the straight facts about the odds. Most people appreciate honesty, but some are startled that you're being so blunt.

I finally got around to reading Shem's *House of God* recently, and I enjoyed it very much. It's kind of a medical *Animal House*. It was fun, and there's a lot of truth hidden behind all the burlesque, but classifying anesthesiology as a 'no-patient-care' specialty is just ignorance. Surgeons only take care of the strictly mechanical and medical problems. We take care of the patients—the stuff they don't seem to have time for or don't think is important.

Let's see if I can take you through a typical day. I'm up at 4 A.M. and in the hospital somewhere between 5 and 5:15 A.M. I get the OR prepared for anesthesia, with both physical equipment and medications. The patient is usually in the OR by 6:30 A.M. and being prepped. At that point, I start the IVs going, and the patient is completely asleep and ready for surgery by 7:30 A.M. We do surgery all day. I can usually get a half-hour break sometime in the morning and then again in the early afternoon if things are going well. If the patient is not in trouble, a nurse anesthetist will break us out so we can catch our breath and get something to eat. But you can't leave if there is any problem with the patient. Surgery is usually over between 6 and 7 P.M.

After you are out of the OR, which also means you are sure the patients are safely out of anesthesia, then you start checking the list of operative patients for the next day. We have to round on each one, read the chart, examine them, review their medical backgrounds and the surgical plan, and make decisions concerning what type of anesthesia is to be used. As I said before, much of your time in the evenings is spent as a patient advocate. Surgeons don't discuss much with patients. They hardly see them before the surgery; we are the people who explain things. You do your own history and physical because you are interested in different things from the surgeon. You have to know the patient.

I usually get out of the hospital around 9 P.M. if I'm not on call. If I'm totally wiped out, I tumble into bed after a few words with my wife because I have to get up at 4 A.M. and start all over. If I have any energy left, I spend some time with her. It's very tough for her now. She has an accounting background, but the company she was working for went Chapter 11, so she's unemployed and has nothing to do. She has all this unstructured time on her hands, and I'm pretty unavailable. She still can't understand why I have to give other people my attention when she needs me. It's a bad stressor—no doubt about it. She hasn't fully adjusted yet. It's probably the reason that more engagements and marriages break up in medicine than in anything else.

And then, in addition, I'm on call about one night in four. How busy you are depends on which hospital you're assigned to at the time. At the University Hospital, you can count on being up all night. One advantage is that the day after you've been on call, you have off. You're not allowed to work or administer any anesthesia. Maybe it's a state law. I don't know. I used to go home and go right to bed, but as I've become more frustrated by the lack of personal time, I tend to push myself and not go to bed. I try to do things I want to do and do things with my wife.

It's funny though, when you're on at night, there's not much difference between 2 P.M. and 2 A.M. Your job is pretty much the same, and the stresses are the same. There are no windows in the OR, and there's no feeling of night or day, and you forget what time it is. You try not to think about it. You're either wired or tired. If I talk to my wife on the phone, I ask her what it's like out in the world. You can sort of tell when the new day is starting by seeing new people come in. That's the only sign you have.

You're not only doing emergency cases at night but a lot of organ transplants. Because they take so long, they tend to monopolize OR time. If all transplants were scheduled during the day, nobody else could do any surgery. Many transplants start at 6 P.M. and go all night. A liver transplant can take anywhere from 8 to 30 hours—and you are also controlled by when the organs become available. Sometimes, you can't sit around, especially with hearts. You have to be ready to go when the organ is available.

As you can see, there's a helluva price to pay for doing this kind of work, but I'm not having any second thoughts, I really couldn't be happy doing anything else. I was a physiology major in college and then worked as a cell biologist for a few years and then got interested in medicine, so I'm a few years behind my classmates. But I had plenty of chance to think it over before making the move, and now I look forward to coming to work every morning despite the 4 A.M. wakeup.

In medical school, I liked most things, but there are some specialties where you feel the patients are too sick or too hopeless and you feel you're not doing very much for them. Conversely, there are some where you feel that the problems you'll be dealing with aren't significant enough to warrant your time. I guess it boils down to what you find stimulating and what you think gives you the best chance of balancing your personal and professional lives.

There's a lot of physiology in anesthesiology so you know what you're doing. Much of the time, your decisions are governed by hard numbers. In internal medicine, you are often feeling your way around, and it may be weeks or months before you see any results from what you are doing. In anesthesiology, it's all out in front of you in a few hours, and you have the satisfaction of knowing you did a good job immediately.

Also, it's fun—it's kind of risky. You feel very much in control, but you know that if you're not right on the ball, the patient can die on you or get terrible complications. It's like driving a racing car—it's exciting—controlled and fast.

Now that I'm a senior resident, I'm on my own a lot, though I do have to check things out with an attending. At night, after I've seen the preops, I call the attending I'll be working with the next morning and tell him what I've found and what decisions I've made about anesthesia. Usually, they go along with me now, and if they don't, we discuss it and they tell me why. In the OR, one attending will circulate between three senior residents, but with the first-year people, they have an attending in the room at all times. You can always get help if you need it. Sometimes, it's information. Sometimes you're just having trouble getting an airway into a patient. That's not a science; it's an art. You can't sit there and figure it out if you're in trouble. You just call an attending to see if he or she can do it. Or sometimes, there's a sudden drop in blood pressure and you need four hands instead of two.

A good attending is someone who gets the best out of you without intimidating you, without looking down on you or being supercritical. That's a rare person, much less a rare physician. We have over 30 attendings, but no more than 5 or 6 meet those criteria. Most have lost their insight into the pressures of what it's like to be a resident and don't understand what you're living through. There's a skill to teaching a resident who's now faced with an overwhelming amount of information that's completely new and has to be absorbed quickly. I don't know whether it's the stress or the rush of work, but most attendings don't have the patience to stay with you long enough while you learn.

I've watched many of them now as they become bitter and resentful. I have a lot of problems now with what I see as my role models—lots of people that I don't want to become like as I get older. They seem to resent the loss of their personal life and loss of control over things. Medicine is very demanding, and these people seem to have underestimated what it takes in terms of time and emotions. A lot of them say they are locked into medicine at this point and can't make a change but would never do it again if they had the chance.

Of course, we have to interact with the surgical attendings, too. They're a different breed. They want to operate. In the old days, before modern anesthesia, the surgeon ran the operating room. The anesthesiologist carried out the surgeon's orders. Now, it's different. There's an operative side to the OR and an anesthesia side. They do their job and we do ours. There are very few confrontations. If a surgical resident or a junior surgical attending tries to tell me what to do, I don't pay a lot of attention. Once in a while, a senior surgeon will try it. I don't argue. I just call my attending and let him or her handle it.

It's no myth about the heavy use of drugs in our specialty. We've already lost one member of our resident group for that reason. It's a combination of easy access and personality. The people who tend to do it are experimenters and like to fool around—and they're addicted. I'm not sure about this, but I think drugs are being used both at home and in the hospital. That's what makes it scary. That's addiction; you can no longer differentiate home from work.

Every group is involved: house officers, attendings, and nurses. We talk about it, but not as much as we should. There's a certain amount of looking the other way. Even when a problem is recognized, they say, 'Get better' or send the person away for a month to some detox program and expect him or her to come back and function as a new person in 30 days. I think that's unrealistic and uncaring.

Basically, I'm personally satisfied with the residency, and I don't see the need for much change. There are a lot of petty, little things—you feel like you're giving your soul to a hospital and when they soak you $80 a month for a parking place so you can come in at five in the morning and they're only paying you $20,000 a year, it's pretty irritating.

Where am I headed in the future? I guess I'm going to pursue a pain fellowship. I wouldn't want to do that full time. I will always want to spend a few days a week in the OR. But it would be good to be the medical director of a pain center. This is a pretty new subspecialty. Right now, there's a lot of chiropractic and acupuncture stuff going on in that area. One reason I like the idea is that it will give me some of my own patients and more direct patient contact. That's the thing I miss the most.

▲   ▲   ▲

There were several threads running through this interview that repeated themselves in other interviews with anesthesiology house officers. Although these were sometimes interwoven, I believe it is possible to tease them apart and look at them separately.

First, there was the business of self-image. I detected a kind of defensive posture in relation to surgeons. As Dr. R. pointed out, he was chagrined by the accusation that his specialty is not concerned with patient care. He aggressively pointed out that it was he and his colleagues who took care of surgical patients while surgeons were busy cutting things out or rearranging them.

The image of the powerful surgeon as the ship captain standing on the bridge giving orders while others dash around doing his or her bidding made these young people chafe. They were concerned that this was both the public and the professional image of their specialty and hastened to assure me that, although this may have been true in the past, high-technology techniques for monitoring of patients' status have changed all of that.

As another house officer told me, "Part of it, I think, is that you can do a wonderful case on an extremely sick patient with a wonderful outcome, and all they care about is how their bandage looks or their incision, and you kind of walk away like the forgotten doctor. That's not so good for your ego. Remember the *Newsweek* photo when Reagan was shot, and they showed all the doctors in the OR and everybody was named but the guy at the head of the table, who was the anesthesiologist and who probably saved Reagan's life—the forgotten doctor? It's a low-profile specialty. You just don't get very many pats on the back when, in fact, you are more responsible for the patient's welfare than almost anybody else. When things go wrong, you get hell. When things go right, you don't get the credit."

This undertone of mixed feelings toward surgery and surgeons ran through all of the interviews. Each of the house officers whom I interviewed in this specialty had seriously entertained the idea of becoming a surgeon at many points in their careers. I got the sense that, in some instances, they had relinquished this goal incompletely and were left with certain lingering yearnings.

Virtually all of the house officers interviewed as a part of this book told me that if I really wanted to know the facts about alcohol and substance abuse, I should talk to the anesthesiology residents. So, when that opportunity presented itself, I pursued the question. Each of them told me without hesitation that drug abuse was most serious not only among anesthesiology house officers but among nursing personnel and attending physicians in this specialty. The simplest explanation has to do with easy access to mind-altering drugs. The house officers were not satisfied with this explanation, however. Furthermore, as Dr. R. pointed out, many were not convinced that sufficient attention was being paid to this problem by those in authority (until it was too late) because the seriousness of the situation was being underestimated. Perhaps this "looking the other way" gave a kind of tacit approval to junior personnel.

Another house officer told me,

▼   ▼   ▼

You know, one of the theories about why drug abuse is so rampant in this field has to do with our isolated, Lone Ranger, bottom-guy-on-the-surgical-totem-pole image. I agree that it is rampant, but I don't agree with the theory. The fascinating thing to me is that most of the people who do it are the best people, not the worst ones. I've asked myself if this is just another one of their experiences, like another challenge—like they are so good, they have to try this too. Or is it boredom or stress? I don't have the answer any more than anybody else, but I can tell you this: the day I pick up a syringe is the day I quit my job.

How can people do this to themselves? We lost one of our best residents not long ago. He OD'd. One nurse was found on the bathroom floor unconscious with a bottle of inhalational anesthesia in her hand. Some of these guys, you know what's going on but you deny it and don't really face it, and then you find out afterward that they are in a rehab program. You can bet that will never happen to me. I didn't get into this field for that. I told you it was a lifestyle choice—I mean, getting off at a reasonable hour, signing out the patients to somebody else, spending time with my wife, exercising, socializing, having a personal life.

▲   ▲   ▲

Obviously, the question of substance abuse was seen as being much more complex and much more pervasive than can be explained by the simpleminded statement, "Well, anesthesia people can pick all that stuff up like peanuts or popcorn."

As mentioned above, a related theme that constantly emerged from this and other interviews was the picture of the anesthesiologist as Lone Ranger.

One resident told me,

▼   ▼   ▼

The other thing is that there is kind of an isolation. There is no peer group. We don't see each other. We only see one attending at a time, but there is no peer support group and no peer teaching like there is in other specialties. In radiology, you sit around and look at films together. In medicine, you go on rounds, but we do pretty much everything alone. We might have one conference a week or something, sitting around the table, so there is very little social interaction in the group.

You miss out on the peer teaching and the peer support system in anesthesia. It's zero. Even when you are an intern, it's you and the attending; you never really work with the senior residents.

▲   ▲   ▲

And yet another resident, while observing the aloneness of the anesthesiologist, also gave me some hint concerning what was attractive about the work:

▼   ▼   ▼

In anesthesiology, you are really a loner. You don't like other people taking care of your patient. This is one reason we take so few breaks in the OR. It's just you and the patient. But it's also a good place to hide your incompetence at the same time, because nobody really knows what you're doing, and you can get away with almost anything just so you don't kill the patient. Or you have gone into it because you don't speak the language and you don't have to deal with patients.

At another hospital we work at, those people are up there alone, and who is to tell them what to do or that they sometimes don't know what they are doing? Many of them speak such poor English that you wouldn't know how to tell them anyway. And if you are working in a setting where you have residents to do the preop assessments, you don't even have to talk to the patient before the operation.

▲   ▲   ▲

Still another resident said, in connection with the aloneness, "If I'm doing my own case and it's a big case, I don't want somebody coming in for 20 minutes while I eat or go to the bathroom and changing the game plan. I know what I'm doing and he doesn't know the case. Some patients, as they start to wake up, their blood pressure goes up. With some, it starts to go down because they get vagal, and if that happens when your relief is sitting there, he may give the patient something unnecessary that screws up the works when actually what happened didn't really need anything. You have this feeling of protection for the patient and wanting to do the best for the patient, so there are days when I would be in the OR at the University Hospital from a quarter to seven to a quarter to seven. That takes a pretty big bladder."

This sense of being in control of the patient's physiology, of "running the patient"—the heart, the lungs, even the gastrointestinal tract, if necessary—seems to compensate in some measure for the loss of autonomy experienced in giving up the surgical role.

Remember that what characterizes all of the specialists in this section is that, for the most part, they do not have their own patients; rather, they support the efforts of other physicians. This sense of decreased patient contact, which for most physicians was one of the important attractions of medicine in the first place, was perhaps less characteristic of anesthesiology than of radiology or clinical pathology. Nevertheless, it was an issue with many house officers and attendings. Dr. R. whom we heard from at the beginning of the chapter, planned to handle some of his sense of loss by pursuing a pain fellowship and then spending a good part of his time working in a pain center. This would permit him to have his own patients.

In some instances, the conscious choice of anesthesiology appeared to be an escape from the responsibility for long-term patient involvement. The work was attractive because the results were immediate, patient care was circumscribed both by act and by the clock, and final responsibility for care rested with another physician. Some did not view anesthesiology as a specialty with reduced patient contact. In this context, the nature of the practice did not present any problem. As one resident told me, "In contrast to other hospital-based specialties, I think we have a lot of patient contact and are very heavily involved in patient care, so I don't miss anything being in this specialty. I think we give the best possible care to patients and, in many ways, take care of the patients a lot better than the surgeons do, most of whom are doing mechanical tasks anyway."

All of the house officers whom I interviewed stressed the special rhythm of work in anesthesiology. The word *pace* was used repeatedly.

Dr. R. referred to the fun of it, the sense of riskiness. He talked about the need to be on the ball at all times, about the patients' ability to die on him without warning. He compared it to driving a racing car, exciting but controlled and fast.

In describing his experience at the OB hospital, another resident said,

▼   ▼   ▼

It's different from most specialties. You have to think and act at the same time. In medicine or psychiatry, you often have hours or even days to think about what to do or the results of what you have done. In surgery, you usually have minutes. In anesthesiology, you usually have seconds.

An emergency cesarean section is the most strenuous and stressful thing in OB, and I don't think I react to stress like most people. It takes an awful lot to get me stressed. Severe stress at the OB hospital is a woman who has severe toxemia of pregnancy, and all of a sudden, her baby's heart rate slows down, and she just ate two Big Mac's before she came in the hospital, and she comes in and we are expected to have her asleep and let them cut the baby out like in 45 seconds or something.

Remember that she can have bad problems with [blood] clotting time, and her blood pressure is 190 over 120. You have to put those people to sleep because you don't have time for regional anesthesia. It takes too long and there is no time for that. You do a rapid-sequence induction, keep a lot of pressure on their neck, keep a lot of suction canisters ready. You intubate her and have it done quickly by a very skillful person. You have to worry about her blood pressure not getting too high. Some of these people have hidden aneurysms that can blow up on them. We had a case a few weeks ago where the woman died from a cerebral hemorrhage, but we were able to save the baby. It's tough because you have to worry about a young, healthy mom and a baby who are suddenly in a great deal of trouble. You are usually not on your own when something like this happens. Usually, there are several people around to help you, including an attending and maybe another resident and some nurse anesthetists, and while you are doing one thing, somebody is taking care of other things. It's really tough to try to do all those at once, but if it happens in the middle of the night and somebody needs to be put to sleep very quickly and you're the only one there, at least in the immediate vicinity, you have to go ahead with it.

The thing about anesthesiology is that the hotter things get and the more stressful things seem to everybody else in the room, the cooler the person at the head of the table has to be. That defines the fine line between somebody who might be very smart but clinically not very good in anesthesia. You've got to be able to stay calm and cool, or you miss things and make mistakes. You've got to be able to think and act at the same time.

In the 30 seconds that you are doing an induction on somebody, an awful lot of things can happen, and you have to watch it all. Things do go wrong and you have to hope that it's not because of pilot error.

▲   ▲   ▲

In Part VI, we will have several things to say about the significance, for better or worse, of the interactions between house officers and attending physicians. However, there is a specific feature in this area for anesthesiology that we must underscore at this point. This brings us once more to the special importance of surgical attendings to anesthesiologists. They work in surgical operating rooms together. At times, house officers are administering anesthesia while surgery is being performed by senior surgical attendings. The delicate balance between the operating side of the patient's care and the anesthesia side must be maintained if the patient is to stand the best chance of favorable outcome. Yet, conflicts and fundamental differences of opinion about proper care may arise. When this occurs, the anesthesiology house officer must depend on his or her own attending to "run interference," or to serve as a buffer zone in the conflict. Generally, this does not occur in other specialties, even other hospital-based specialties such as radiology and clinical pathology.

Dr. R., whose interview appears at the beginning of this chapter, did not seem to have much problem in this area. However, some of his peers did. For instance, one told me, "One of the parts of anesthesia that upsets me more than anything is if you have an attending who is a wimp, he can get pushed around by the surgeon, who may want things done a certain way even if it isn't the right way and best for the patient. Your attending will sort of cave in, and then you are in the middle and you just have to go along with it. You can't get caught in that conflict. That happens more than you know because some of these guys just won't stand up for what they know is right in the face of an intimidating surgeon. That really bothers me. Usually, these things revolve around the fact that the surgeon or the OB guy doesn't really know beans about physiology and is arguing out of ignorance, and the anesthesiologist, who does know physiology and hemodynamics and so on and has the facts, just doesn't stick up for what is best for the patient. I really get upset about that."

In a more dramatic episode, another reported,

▼   ▼   ▼

A case at the University Hospital I won't forget for a long time was a man of about 50. He was a postoperative osteogenic sarcoma and had been supposedly successfully treated with chemotherapy. He was now being admitted for a heart transplant! I was on cardiac at the time, and it turned out to be my case. On preop assessment, he turned out to have very high cardiac pulmonary resistance, which is one of the contraindications to cardiac transplant, but for some reason, they decided to go ahead anyway. Number one, they chose the wrong patient. Number two, they chose the wrong procedure. The topper was that, after we had put the patient to sleep, a nurse came running into the OR to say that the lab reports had been wrong and that this was not a good tissue match for an organ transplant for this patient. They had already taken out the patient's heart and were putting the last sutures in the donor heart. Now, we were faced with an acute rejection of this heart in a patient who already had a life-threatening disease.

We kept him alive for a few days, and then, I had to be the anesthesia person again when they took the first heart out and put in a second one a week later. These are the occasions when anesthesiologists should not act like wimps but should stand up to surgery and refuse to give anesthesia to a patient like that.

▲   ▲   ▲

Again, this critical relationship between house officer and attending emerged as the fulcrum around which training revolved. In one form or another, this pivotal interaction was described by almost all house officers as the single most important force determining the outcome of their training experience. It seems that, in anesthesiology, this took on special meaning, as the house officers had to confront the demands of the surgeons, with whom they worked on a daily basis.

Chapter 14

RADIOLOGY

Dr. M. is a 28-year-old fourth-year resident in radiology. He is married and the father of two small children. His wife is a full-time homemaker. He appeared exactly on time for his appointment, carrying a soft drink in a large paper cup. As he sat down, he withdrew a sandwich wrapped in wax paper from the pocket of his jacket with his free hand and proceeded to manage both deftly while talking with me. Shortly, the aroma of garlic wafted through the office, accompanied by the audible rumbling of my stomach, as I had not had time for lunch. He paid no attention to either the olfactory or the auditory distractions as he happily demolished his own lunch. He was not the picture of sartorial splendor: his button-down shirt was badly pilled at the collar, his black knit tie was askew, and his corduroy slacks were rumpled and baggy.

▼   ▼   ▼

I got into this specialty by a process of elimination. I didn't like internal medicine because I don't have the right temperament for that kind of work or working with those people; they are very nerdy, too intense and obsessional. They feel like they have to know everything. If one little lab finding is abnormal, they are likely to repeat all the studies because they are so afraid of missing something. My impulse is to repeat that one test and see what you get the second time. Maybe the other thing I didn't like about it was the intensity. You are working with a population of patients who are usually very sick for a long period of time. A lot of them die, and you have to deal with that inside yourself and with their families—and they are always making demands on you, some of which you can't meet.

It's one thing to do an angiogram on a patient who has a tumor. I can feel bad about it and chat with him but I won't see him again. I don't have the struggle of trying to cope with this hopeless disease in this man who just retired at 65 years and was planning to move to Arizona or California with his wife—and now all their plans are out the window and he'll be dead in a year or so. I don't want to work in a specialty like that.

I also considered surgery because I like doing procedures, but the life-style turned me off. There is no space in their lives for anything else and no real opportunity for family life, which is a high priority for me. I wanted a specialty where there would be some personal time and yet you could feel that you were making a real contribution to the diagnosis and care of the patient. I had some hesitation about radiology because of the low level of patient contact, but I finally decided that there are enough procedures like ultrasound and angiography that have some patient contact to make it a reasonable trade-off.

At one point, I considered switching to emergency medicine or critical-care medicine, but I was afraid either of early burnout or long-term boredom. You either have the endless stress of an ICU, or you're working in some ER taking care of one sore throat or earache or headache or bellyache after another with people who don't have their own doctors. I would go looney tunes doing that.

What I miss even more than the patient contact is the interaction and team aspects of work in specialties like medicine and surgery. In radiology, you're kind of a Lone Ranger most of the time. It's pretty isolating. Some-times, you sit and read 100 or 150 flat plates and dictate into a machine, and you don't see another human being for hours. You do have some interaction with the surgical house officers because they come down, look at the films with you, and discuss them. There's a real interchange. The medicine resi-dents are more likely to come down, look at the films themselves, ask a few questions, and disappear.

I sound like I have some mixed feelings about my choice of specialty, but basically, it's right for me. It will give me what I want over the long run. What is most attractive, in spite of what I've said, is, well, you get this flat plate of the abdomen and it looks like there is something suspicious in one of the kidneys, so then you do an ultrasound study and, by golly, there is a mass in the upper pole that looks fairly extensive. So then, you can do a CT scan and get a clear definition of the dimensions and spread of the mass. And then, before the surgeons go in, you do an angiogram because they will want to know the vascular supply to the mass, what it has encroached on, whether it has spread into the major blood vessels, and so on. So you have supplied for the surgeon a complete picture of what he or she is facing, what risks there are, what the problems are going to be, what the anatomy is. That is an enormous contribution to good patient care that wasn't possible 10 years ago.

My current assignment happens to be angiography. As you might guess, I enjoy it because I like to perform procedures. You sort of feel like a surgeon. There you are in a room with the patient who gets draped and skin-prepped; then I must anesthetize the skin, cut down on the artery, and insert a needle, through which is extended a pliable wire, which I must feed through the system to the right place as I observe the fluoroscope. Then, over the wire is fed a catheter, through which the contrast die is injected. It's a delicate procedure, but it's low-risk. It's satisfying to do because you get immediate results, and it can be extremely helpful to the surgeon.

My typical day right now consists of getting in about 8:00 A.M. and doing one angiography after another. You can do only about four or five a day because they take so long. I'm generally finished about 5:30 P.M., and I can go home just when some of the other residents are warming up for evening rounds and working up new admissions. We take a lot of kidding about this, but I'm feeling more and more comfortable about our role and our ability to make important contributions to the patient's care.

Of course, if you're on call, it's different, but that's only about once a month. Then you're up all night because this is such a big trauma center and because we do so many organ transplants. Once a month is a piece of cake, though.

As you can see, this doesn't qualify as a terribly stressful residency compared to some others. When people say that physicians and house officers are among the worst drug and alcohol abusers, I must be blind. I see zero in our department. Maybe it's because I'm married and out of that social swim, or maybe I'm just naive, but I haven't seen anybody come in looking hungover or spacy.

Outside of the relative lack of patient contact, I think the toughest stress we have to face has to do with the endless body of information you have to master. Not only are there rapid advances being made in every phase of radiology which you're supposed to keep abreast of, but you've got to have a good working knowledge of most specialties and disease states so you have some sense of what you're looking at on the films and you can discuss the disease process intelligently with the individual who referred the patient. This data base is a bottomless pit, and it's a very humbling process to attempt to master.

Therefore, I try to get in very early every morning to read for 90 minutes before the patients start arriving. I also keep using the department's teaching file of films, and I go to as many of the clinical conferences as I can. When I have to present at these, I don't do very well because I have trouble remembering all the information about a case and integrating it. I choke up a bit in front of a large group, especially if there's an attending leading the conference who's kind of intimidating.

There are a lot of attendings who don't treat you like a colleague but more like a student. You lead sort of a schizophrenic existence. You go home and you're a father and a husband and so on, and you come to the hospital and you have this layer upon layer of superiors and teachers telling you what to do all day long—evaluating and judging you—with a great deal of power over your life. After all these years, you get a little sick of it.

Maybe you wouldn't mind so much if most of the attendings also spent a lot of time with you pointing out things you may have missed and helping you get a deeper understanding of what you're looking at. Unfortunately, I'll bet less than a fourth of the attendings are like that. Most don't treat you as a colleague and don't place much emphasis on teaching. Their priorities are elsewhere, of necessity. They have to bring in money through grants, and they have to turn out publishable research—and it's the rare person who can do it all. You want to please the staff you are working with, and that's hard enough at our age because it makes you feel subservient. If you have an attending who's distant and unfriendly and has his or her mind on other things, it puts you down and grates on your nerves.

I find I'm really enjoying this interview. It's personal time for me. I don't get a chance to do something like this. I'm either meeting demands at home or at work, and there is rarely any time to sit down and think or go over where I am or what I want to do. Nobody ever sits with me and talks about me and what I'm doing. It's kind of frustrating because no time is your own. I don't even have time to exercise or read for pleasure.

If I were the chairman, I'd try to change the reward system so that the best teachers would get more goodies. I'm selfishly afraid that we are going to lose the four or five people we do have who are genuinely interested in the residents. Maybe they'll get too frustrated in trying to advance themselves and they'll move into private practice or other systems. Those people tend not to be squeaking wheels and don't get pushy about being advanced. They enjoy clinical work and teaching, and they don't look like superstars, but to the residents, they're worth their weight in gold.

What keeps me going is my family and our thoughts of the future. You're probably going to laugh after what I've said about how fed up I am with being a student, but after my residency, I'm planning to take a a two-year fellowship in neuroradiology. The field is getting pretty saturated with radiologists, and you have to subspecialize if you're going to be a marketable commodity.

My wife and I are very much looking forward to the future. She's aware that this is a rather lucrative field with lots of good personal time. We just need to get through the next few years and the financial strain of being a house officer with a family and no other source of income; but we'll make it, and then things will be a lot better. I realize I'm not a superstar, but I'm competent and I will do a good job. And I'll try to find a good balance between my personal and professional lives.

I'm not interested in working for somebody or being an employee after all this. I'm going into practice, and I want to be a partner, a full partner, not taking a lot of orders. I will have spent too many years mastering all of this to be taking orders from anybody.

▲   ▲   ▲

Because of radiology's basic characteristics as a hospital-based specialty, many of the same themes inevitably emerged in this interview that we saw in the interviews with anesthesiology house officers. Concerns about the status and future of the specialty, issues relating to the amount of direct patient contact, and matters of isolation from other professionals were important.

The choice of radiology because of the lifestyle it offers and the opportunity to integrate the intellectual rigors of hard science, especially those of physics and mathematics, with clinical knowledge about human disease was emphasized by all these house officers. Indeed, as Dr. M. pointed out, sometimes the almost infinite number of facts that the radiologist must attempt to master may also be the most stressful aspect of the specialty.

Another house officer stated eloquently,

▼   ▼   ▼

One of the toughest things in this specialty is that there is no limit to the data you have to master. In addition to all the rapid changes in different modalities of diagnosis, like CT scanning, plane-field radiographs, ultrasound, nuclear medicine, and magnetic-resonance imaging, you have to know a great deal about almost any disease because you have to be ready to interpret what you see as an ongoing disease process with all the different specialists. For instance, in medical school, you don't learn much about these complex congenital abnormalities in babies and young children, but when you are on pediatric radiology, you run into them all the time, and you have to know what they are and be able to discuss them in detail with the pediatricians. It's the same in OB/GYN, in cardiology, in neurosurgery, and so on.

There may be no other specialty where you have to master so much information. It's kind of overwhelming. You have to be able to work with other clinicians and understand what they need. Sometimes, they don't even ask the right questions, so you have to know the questions better than they do. You also have to have a good knowledge of anatomy, physiology, pathology, and physics.

There's a kind of paradox in this. Because of the growing body of information you have to know, more and more radiologists are subspecializing, like in pediatrics or neuroradiology—you just can't know all this. On the other hand, if you have any interest in patient contact, you sort of feel out of it. You feel like you have to know an enormous amount of medicine, and in other ways, you feel less and less like a practicing physician.

▲   ▲   ▲

This last point is important also. Many house officers pointed out that the growing pressure to know more and more about less and less in their specialty compelled them to subspecialize too early in their careers. This might prevent them from achieving the kind of breadth that a genuinely seasoned clinical teacher needs in order to serve as an excellent role model for succeeding generations of trainees.

Dr. R. was certainly not the only house officer who thanked me for providing an opportunity to express his views in detail about his or her training experience, but few did it as eloquently as he did. All of the house officers in the hospital-based specialties, however, seemed to point to this as one of the least desirable aspects of their training. Many thought of subspecializing in areas that would permit them to function more as team members, but sometimes this was not feasible or at least not practical. Some wondered whether they had selected these specialties because they enjoyed isolation.

Another aspect that emerged frequently had to do with a sense that the functions and contributions of the specialty were not truly understood by other physicians. Perhaps this even took the form of intentional misuse or exploitation at times.

In describing his typical day, one radiology resident said, "By late afternoon, you are getting calls about add-on's or emergency scans that come in and have to be done at the last minute. Lots of emergencies are not emergencies at all. People just want them done quickly. They don't understand that CT scans that are done in the evening or the middle of the night may not have the same quality because you don't have a full staff present. Often, it's much better to delay until regular hours. We try to explain that, but some attendings want what they want *now*. Some residents are not above lying and will call almost anything an emergency. They get you in to do things in the middle of the night so they are ahead of the game the next day. They think radiology residents don't work hard enough anyway. There's nothing much you can do about that. They just deny it if you confront them."

A corollary is that, apparently, radiology can become deadeningly routine in some large, highly specialized centers. The radiology resident may start to feel that he or she is simply a mechanical tail being wagged by a large dog over which she or he has no control. Dr. J., a third-year radiology house officer, described this feeling as follows:

▼   ▼   ▼

On the gastrointestinal rotation, this is much better at other hospitals than it is at the University Hospital because it is a large transplant center. This has made the GI assignment too heavy on posttransplant liver studies. You keep on looking at the same thing over and over again. The surgeons need to follow the patient for this reason, but it gets like a treadmill for the residents because you are seeing so many patients with the same thing and there is nothing new to learn for you. Instead of feeling like a doctor, you get to feel like a technician after a while. Now, even a large part of the ultrasound and CT assignment is consumed with transplant work, which also gets to be very routine. For instance, some of the kidney transplants get an ultrasound every day. The transplant teams have gotten so large and diffuse that some of them don't even know the names of the patients, and they may even order studies that are not needed. Then you are surprised that you have spent an hour or two doing something that they don't really care about. This is very frustrating, sometimes especially because you get the feeling that you are not helping the patient or contributing to the care.

In general, I've been getting the feeling that what I do for these patients doesn't make a lot of difference. Maybe it's because so many of them, especially liver patients, are not doing well lately and are getting into a lot of trouble—like, they will ask you to do an angiogram because they think the hepatic artery is blocked, and you do it and there is no donor anyway for the patient, so the patient dies. It's a terrible Catch-22 for the patient. If they suppress their immune systems to the point where they don't reject the organs, then they are open to anything that comes along by way of infection, and they don't seem to be able to get a handle on that. This whole transplant service is starting to double up our time. Sometimes we just feel like an extension of them. Lots of the residents are feeling irritated and overwhelmed by it.

This is part of the fun of getting out of the University Hospital and rotating to some of the other four or five hospitals where you can do more general radiology, which prepares you for practice, instead of the highly specialized unusual stuff or the flood of transplant work you have to do at the University. Sometimes you really worry that you are not spending enough of your time on things that are really relevant to the future. You could spend years working in a community hospital in a radiology department and never see a patient who had a transplant. When we go to a community hospital on a GI rotation, we see gall bladders, gastric ulcers, possibility of colon cancer—that kind of stuff.

▲   ▲   ▲

On balance, however, the house officers with whom I spoke seemed more satisfied with their plight than not. They seemed to be receiving from their training those rewards that were most important to them, and their choice of specialty remained firm despite its unusual stresses and pressure.

BIBLIOGRAPHY

Miller RE: The stresses of training: A preceptor's perceptions. American
    Roentgan Ray Society 137:1088–1090, 1981.

Chapter 15

CLINICAL PATHOLOGY

Dr. H. is a 27-year-old third-year pathology resident. He has been married for six months to a lab technician. She is a native in the city, but he had migrated east from Wisconsin, where he went to school. He has a quick, boyish smile and, in fact, appears several years younger than his stated age. He was very casually dressed in a plain sport shirt, chinos, and scuffed loafers—all topped off with a thick, shiny helmet of blue-black hair. As he became involved in the flow of the interview, he smiled much less frequently and grew more intense, expounding with almost no prompting on a variety of subjects related to his choice of specialty and to his particular training program. At these points in the interview, his facial expression changed, and his image emerged as more mature, more age-appropriate.

▼   ▼   ▼

Pathology residents are not given the same level of autonomy and responsibility that residents in other specialties get. In internal medicine, say, you have your own clinical patients. You can check with the attending when you need help and he or she may sign off on your charts or something. But these are your patients and you take care of them. In pathology, you have no such responsibility, at least not in a university center. The program is five years long, and although you learn more and more as you go along, you never do anything by yourself. A chief resident in pathology basically has no more responsibility than an intern.

If you've been a chief resident and then you come on the faculty, suddenly you can go from no responsibility to total responsibility in 24 hours. There's nothing in between. Therefore, the stresses of the residency are quite different from other specialties. You're always a student until you finish. You never feel scared, like you're in a different role from when you were a med student. You're not making life-or-death decisions in emergencies and so on. That part of it is easy.

The transition comes five years later, when you go from chief resident to attending, and you suddenly find there is no one to back you up anymore. It's kind of funny to watch a recently graduated chief resident on the first few cases. They can overreact with the most routine things that they've seen a thousand times before. You hear them muttering to themselves, 'Dammit, I've never seen anything like this before in a case of cirrhosis of the liver. What does this mean? Why did this happen to me?' They start acting as if this is the first case ever like this and they've got it. They start looking at every cell on the slide and sweating.

During the first year of training, you work your fanny off physically, but actually, there is very little thinking that you have to do. It's entirely non-academic. It's more administrative. You don't need an M.D. to do what a first-year resident does. You have to be sure things are done on schedule: making sure that the slides are prepared in time for review, that drafts of reports are ready for sign-off by the attending. You get rewarded for being well organized and for knowing what you can say to each attending and when—which ones you can joke with, and when to shut up. You just sort of mark time to get through that first year because you know you're going to be working from 7:30 A.M. until late in the evening most nights, that your opinion about cases won't count for much, that you're very vulnerable to criticism—and that it doesn't matter much anyway because nobody's life or welfare depends on your being right or wrong.

I know there are rumors about house officers' relying on drugs or alcohol to handle the stresses of training. I don't think we have any users. I've never seen any of our people under the weather or unable to function. You're not in the middle of the fray. You don't have the pressures of a medical or surgical resident. It's more plodding through one body of facts after another, more like going to medical school again than being a real doctor.

The only way it can be different is if you train in a community hospital residency instead of a university. But that's kind of a Catch-22. In a community hospital, you don't see a broad enough spectrum of material over time to get really good training. Also, you can run into the flip side of what we've got here. Instead of almost no responsibility, you can end up doing all the work with a very perfunctory sign-off by an attending and with very little teaching. And then, when you graduate from a program like that, it's very hard to get a decent job.

My current assignment is in cytology, where you have to learn to read various body fluids and smears for the presence of abnormal cells—like Pap smears, cerebrospinal fluid, urine, the contents of cysts, that kind of thing. You spend a lot of time hitting the books, and they also have a tremendous collection of classical slides that you can study. And as usual, some of the work involves the examination of actual specimens being sent in from the floors and the OR. You do the first write-up of the report, then an attending goes over the whole thing again, including your write-up. He or she usually makes some changes and then does the final sign-off before the report can go out.

In cytology, the basic trick is to learn what is acceptable as within normal limits for each organ system. The bottom line for attendings is that they are faced with calling the shots concerning whether a specimen contains cells that are benign or malignant. But this varies and depends on where the cell came from. A suspicious cell coming from cerebrospinal fluid is likely to be labeled malignant versus the same cell seen in a urine sample, where you would probably call it normal. You have to learn these things or you can cause the patient and the surgeon a lot of grief. You can set off a lot of false alarms.

Recently, they have added another year to the residency, which is optional for us but compulsory for the new people. It is a straight year of research. I don't know if I would mind that so much, but I would hate to have it forced on me. I doubt if I will take it because I don't see myself going into academic pathology. I've thought about it, but I don't like all the politics of a big department. There is too much conflict and too many hassles.

You might think that the power politics involving the top people in a department really wouldn't have much impact on the residents. Don't kid yourself. One of the attendings has a favorite saying: 'When the elephants fight, the grass dies.' What's going on in our department is no big mystery, and it's probably happening in a lot of programs. That's why they added the year of research to the residency. There is an increasing emphasis on the importance of producing original research. The chairman is making it the number one priority. I think that's the privilege of the chairman: to set priorities. But then you get into situations where some of the other senior faculty members may not line up behind the chairman, and the stage is set for conflict. It's like a family, and the residents may either get caught in the cross fire—or lost in the shuffle.

It's as if too much energy is going into resolving the conflict over priorities in the department, so there may not always be enough left over to train the residents the way you would like. It interferes with the efficient transfer of knowledge to us. We meet with the chairman as a group about four times a year, and he does his best to explain the priorities, what's happening, and what's coming next, but that can't alter the basic situation. I don't want to criticize him. I'm sure he's got his hands full. I know I have no idea what problems a chairman struggles with on a daily basis, and I'm sure it's a thankless job. But the net result for us is that training is coming across as a lower priority, so the faculty puts less into it. They know they're going to be more rewarded for getting research grants and publishing in prestigious journals.

I recognize that this process isn't new. I remember lots of teachers in med school who made it clear they didn't want to be there but they had to be and just gave us their canned lectures. Departments want those grants coming in; they lose money on teaching. But after all, what are we there for? I guess great programs are judged by the number of Nobel laureates, not the quality of the residents they turn out. I can live with that—but you don't want to feel like excess baggage.

That's why when I work with a good attending who's invested in training, I treasure him. If he puts himself into my training and my progress, I will work much harder to please him and put out for him. If he's just going through the motions, I pull back and do just the minimum to get by.

I really enjoy patient contact. That's why choosing a specialty was very hard for me. Everyone told me that, if I went into pathology, I would essentially give up direct work with patients for the rest of my life. The trouble was that I truly loved pathology, and in the end, that took over. Besides, I watched what they call patient contact in a specialty like internal medicine, and I wasn't all that impressed with it. It was sort of 'Hi, Mrs. Jones. How are you this morning? Everything okay? Good! See you tomorrow.' That's not what I call patient contact. I wanted something more intensive than that. Psychiatry appealed to me, but I thought I would have to go into academics to do it right, and I don't think I'm cut out for academic medicine, so I would have ended up in an office listening all day to somebody's marital problems, or about their depression because their mother died, or working with some adolescent with a personality disorder.

In the end, it was pathology. I don't think pathology has to be as isolated from patients as it is. It sometimes operates like a black box. Specimens go in and paper comes out, and nobody ever talks. Even attendings in our department don't seem to talk much to the attendings who send in the lab requests, let alone talk to patients. I don't think it really has to be that way.

Pathologists are not only very straight and conservative, they are socially weird. We may attract a lot of people into our specialty who are trying to get away from patient contact and are socially inept. They may not be very good at communicating with other people. You would notice it at a cocktail party. Maybe there's a reason for the black box. I guess it's self-imposed.

I have no regrets about my choice of specialty, but I'm going to practice it differently from the way they do here. I want more interaction with the rest of the clinical staff where I work, and I want to know a lot more about the patient whose microscopic slides I'm looking at. I think I can do a better job that way.

You just have to make up your mind to get up off your ass and get up on the floor and see the patients. Communication is very important. You have to know what kind of information the clinician wants and for what purpose. You can't do that if you stay in the lab.

You have to know when it's important to labor between two diagnoses and when it doesn't matter very much. We spend a lot of time doing that—only to find out later that the clinician really didn't care. The treatment was the same anyway for both diseases. We spend days doing all these special stains, and then we do this special procedure on the specimen, and then another one, and then we find the patient is already under treatment and halfway out of the hospital—and a whole week has gone by before the piece of paper leaves the black box.

▲   ▲   ▲

Once more, as in the case of anesthesiology and radiology, clinical pathology offered its own particular problems and assets to the house officer. Most notably, and for reasons that may not always have been apparent to the outsider, the clinical pathologist in training was given very little responsibility regardless of his or her level of advancement. This meant that the transition from trainee to staff was a sudden and often chain-yanking experience.

Dr. H., whose words you have just read, was uncomfortable with this enforced dependency, which often extends to age 30 and beyond. Although most trainees understood the reasons intellectually, they rebelled against being treated like a student or a plebe.

Dr. R., who was rather older and had had several years of experience as a laboratory technician before going to medical school, was able to introduce a bit of perspective into the picture, although he, too, was struggling with his status:

▼   ▼   ▼

The way the specialty works, it's the attending who has the actual responsibility for reviewing the findings and signing off on the report, but even as a house officer, you have considerable responsibility. You can do a lot of damage if you mess up. Even in the first year in the autopsy room, you're not just standing around handling the entrails of dead patients. Where you take the sections from each organ, how you mark off the margins of a particular tissue, how the slides are prepared, and how you identify each specimen—all have a considerable impact on what the final diagnostic decisions are. So in this indirect way, you have a good bit of responsibility for what happens. If you're not wide awake in there and you're not thinking every minute, if things get mechanical for you, it's easy to put the wrong label on a cassette or to label a specimen incorrectly, and there's a lot of damage you can inflict that way.

I'm offended by people who think that pathologists don't do very much. We work long hours. Maybe we're not up all night like some specialists, but we work hard and put in our time. I found the first year particularly hard, but it wasn't just the long hours—it was being treated like a plebe again. I was older and more mature than most of the other first-year people, who were straight out of school—they didn't know anything else. But I adjusted. You just go along with it. You swallow it. There's nothing you can do about it anyway.

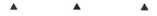

Dr. L., who was a first-year resident, began to experience this lack of responsibility on the part of house officers almost as being a fifth wheel. She wondered whether some of the reasons for the staff's being so protective of its authority had to do with the current practice of defensive medicine. She said,

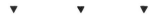

Sometimes, you feel like more of an annoyance to the staff than a help, even though you're doing a lot of work. I know they can do the same thing in half the time we take with a couple of pathology assistants. You feel like a burden because you're slowing the process down. But they slow it down themselves by having to check every detail. They even check the grammar and wording of your reports, and some will take a pen after reading just a few words and strike out a whole page or two and make you do it all over again.

They're so keyed into malpractice issues that they want everything phrased just so to prevent any possible misinterpretation. Some staff are much worse than others about this. They also drill you on questions, sometimes like a catechism. They may not be terribly interested in the case you're doing. They just want you to know the answers to certain questions about that particular disease.

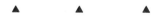

The psychological burdens that go along with assuming trainee status so late in life accompany house officer experience in any specialty, but clinical pathology presented this problem in the extreme. The daily experience for many house officers of assuming the role of husband or wife, mother or father, homeowner and taxpayer for part of the day and relatively impotent student for the rest of it required maximum resiliency. Yet, it may be that many young physicians who entered clinical pathology by nature of their temperament were not the most flexible, easygoing individuals in the world. Remember Dr. H.'s description of his colleagues and teachers as often being "socially weird" or "socially inept." He felt that they might not be very good at communication with other people, and that they enjoyed being in the "black box."

Again, Dr. R. painted the training in a more balanced way: "In pathology training, you are pretty much working with one attending at a time for like a week or so, so whether it's a good experience or an unpleasant one depends on how that person treats you. Some of them are very professional and very autocratic. They want things done exactly their way. Others are more democratic and interact with you more. They will talk to you about your career and your plans and help you along professionally. The whole experience depends on who you are working with at any one time. You don't interact much with anyone else."

But he went on to say, "One of the real problems in training in pathology is that it's possible to slide by as a poor resident because you can always fall back on the attending. They have to sign off on everything; everything gets checked and fixed by them if it's wrong before it leaves the lab. If somebody doesn't pick up the fact that you're not doing very well, it never gets handled, and you can pass through and be rather incompetent. That really bothers me. I don't think pathologists should ever get a job where they're working alone right after training. They should start off as part of a group that has some senior people in it so they can walk down the hall and say, 'What do you think of this?'"

Dr. R. also took greater comfort in his student status. He said, "I like an attending to treat me like a student—somebody who came to learn—not as a servant or a plebe to be harassed. You're sitting there with those people for many hours a day looking through a double-headed microscope. You can only say so much about colon cancer cells after you've looked at three or four slides of them. After a while, you have to talk about other things, and you can tell if they have any interest in you and your future. The really good attendings are not rewarded as much as they should be because they are the genuine teachers, and that's not what you get the most goodies for in the department these days. Very clearly, the first priority is shifting to turning out original research. The ability to train and educate house officers is taking a back seat."

The trainees, in fact, suspected both their teachers and themselves of being happier in a specialty like clinical pathology because they were really not seeking extensive human contact, nor did they want to see a lot of patients directly. Again, Dr. R.'s observations about this phenomenon were:

▼   ▼   ▼

By its very nature, the practice of pathology may lend itself to solo activity—to social isolation, if that's what you want. Some pathologists don't have the best social skills in the world and function best in the lab and away from lots of interpersonal interactions. One of our guys gets in about 5:30 in the morning and makes his resident get in then, too. He gets all of his cases reviewed and finished within a few hours and then spends the rest of the day working in his office. He's a brilliant guy, but he just works better alone. I learned a tremendous amount from him. There's nothing wrong with working alone if that's the way you work best—as long as you do an excellent job. But people generalize this to all pathologists. I guess it's an image problem we have. There are plenty of us who are not like that guy. You get stereotyped, I guess.

I think the whole business of 'patient contact' is one of the most overrated things in the world; it gets overworked by physicians and laypeople also. One of the first questions that a new acquaintance will ask me sometimes is 'Do you have any patients of your own?' It doesn't bother me not to see patients. I don't miss it.

What are you looking for in patients, anyway? Do you want them to say, 'Oh thank you, thank you, thank you, doctor. You're so wonderful. You're a great doctor' and all that kind of stuff? I watch these family practice residents, for instance, who say they want to be involved with people and take care of them through everything, but I've grown suspicious that what they really want to do is control people's lives. Basically, it's a power game to them. They want to be in control of other people.

What it sounds like on the surface is that these patients need you when they get sick or pregnant or their kids get sick. What you have to be cautious about is that you don't end up being dependent on them to feed your ego. There are too many big egos around that need feeding. I don't mind that so much except that these are the very people who go around cutting down others to make themselves feel more important. Those people would be the first ones to say that pathologists are not real doctors.

What they really mean is that pathologists don't have a lot of grateful patients following them around stroking them all the time and telling them how great they are. Maybe as they get older, they'll get to feeling more secure about themselves and they won't have to do that to people anymore.

▲   ▲   ▲

It seems that Dr. R. put his finger on one of the basic motivations in becoming a physician. What he also observed was that, in some, this motivation might reach neurotic proportions, so that the physician needs to feed his or her self-esteem from the praise of doting patients.

In their more sober moments, these young people training in hospital-based specialties felt rather superior to their counterparts in the medical and surgical fields. They saw themselves as making more specific and more measurable contributions to the patients' diagnosis and treatment. As one trainee in clinical pathology said, "The most deadening part of medical school was having to memorize page after page of facts. There was nothing exciting or creative about it. I thought that could easily destroy your brain. It was so different from graduate school, where you had to think. The first two years of medical school were positively insulting for that reason. There was so little emphasis on the mechanisms of disease, so much on what happens and how to recognize and describe it, and not enough on *what* is actually happening and *why*. I guess, in the end, that's what convinced me to go into pathology, which is really the study of the mechanisms of disease—that and the fact that I found most of the treatment procedures boring and ineffective. When you think about it, medicine still doesn't know how to cure most diseases. The best we can do is sort of maintain the patient and keep him or her stabilized."

On that note, I will let these bright and sometimes troubled young people rest their case.

Part IV

THE "GENERAL" SPECIALTIES

The title of this part is, on the face of it, very contradictory. How can one be a generalist and a specialist? This is a neologism of my own making because I could not find any other satisfactory label for this group or trainees. Perhaps many would not place them in the same category, but I believe they belong there because they share some very fundamental features. Most important, both of the specialties described in this part, emergency medicine and family practice, do not focus their attention on any particular age group or any particular organ system of the body or any particular types of disease. In this sense, they are true generalists. They qualify as specialists because their practice requires three years of advanced training. No physician could be expected to practice with expertise in these areas without this training. Hence, the term *specialists* seems justified.

The two groups differ from each other in less important ways than those in which they are similar. The main difference has to do with the fact that family practice physicians provide continuity of care for an entire family group and for most disorders that may appear in the family. Obviously, they are free to refer for more specialized care if they believe the family has developed a disorder that requires more expertise. Emergency medicine physicians, on the other hand, are just that. They may serve the same family members in the same fashion but do not provide continuity of care. Their practice focuses on life-threatening emergencies. They are expert at cardiac resuscitation, at sustaining life in the face of catastrophic injuries, or the sudden rupture of a major blood vessel, or the failure of some other vital organ of the body.

Although these two specialties obviously attract different types of house officers, my own sense is that they are more similar than they are different.

As always, it is better to let these young people speak for themselves.

Chapter 16

EMERGENCY MEDICINE

Dr. W. is a 26-year-old third-year resident in emergency medicine. He is quite young to have arrived at such senior status and looks even younger. He is slight of build and a bit stooped and wears his lank, blue-black hair combed forward over his forehead, Julius Caesar style. His steel-rimmed glasses resembled plexiglass coasters. His hands and feet are disproportionately large for his torso. Although he seemed a bit restless, I did not realize until I listened to the tape of our session how much squirming about he did and how he frequently drummed with his fingers on the metal file cabinet that stood next to his chair. The pockets of his oversized white coat bristled with reflex hammers, pens, lights, stethoscope, and an odd assortment of cards, spiral notebooks, and papers of different sizes and colors held together with paper clips. In addition to the usual beeper clipped to his belt, he carried a large, complicated looking walkie-talkie from which there emitted a variety of buzzing and whirring noises. During the time we spoke, I did not hear a human voice transmitting at any time. Our interview was held during the early evening in the residents' lounge of the Emergency Medicine Center. He insisted that I take the only comfortable chair while he sat on a small molded-plastic bench without a back, explaining that he was tired and didn't want to get too comfortable; rather, he wanted to be alert for the interview. He spoke with surprising poise and self-assurance for someone of his age.

▼   ▼   ▼

I'm just coming off a 36-hour stretch, so I'm a little spacy. I've had two full days in the ER, and I was on call last night. That means accepting continuous radio command for all the city paramedic units.

There are two of us on call every night seven days a week, one on radio command and one on the copter. Many things can be handled by radio, but we have to go out in the city on every cardiac arrest, on any fire that's three alarms or more, on jumpers, on car accidents where there are multiple victims, on hostage situations, and on entrapments where someone has to be extricated from a vehicle.

Last night, there was a cardiac arrest in an outlying section of the city. We had a mobile unit in the area, so they responded quickly. It would have taken me 15 or 20 minutes to get there in our Bronco, so they went and did the immediate work and piled him into the unit, and I met them on the highway halfway between the hospital and the scene. I got into the unit with them, and we rode back to the hospital together. There was also a four-alarm fire last night, and although there were no victims—they all got out in time— you end up treating the firefighters more than the people because of the heat and the fumes.

You can't believe some of the cardiac arrest situations we get into. Last night was a beaut. It turned out to be an 80-year-old guy who had apparently nicked a vein in his leg earlier in the evening. It had just continued to ooze and ooze for hours, but the family didn't call. By the time we knew about it, he had lost a liter or a liter and a half of blood and ended up with a hypovolemic cardiac arrest. The family didn't call for help until he wasn't alert anymore and became short of breath.

When the medics got there, he was lying in bed with his leg hanging over the edge, and the floor was covered with blood. They described how they slid all over the place in blood trying to get him out of the room. They intubated him and established IV access, and then I met them about halfway. They had blood all over their pants from kneeling on the floor while trying to intubate him. The old man was not on any kind of medication. We don't understand why he didn't clot. This morning, we jokingly speculated that maybe the family had been giving him some kind of rat poison with Coumadin or Warfarin in it.

I'm really only kidding about that. What I've learned in emergency medicine is that people will call you if they have a cut on their hand because they can see it. It's real. They may have had tarry stools for four days and think nothing of it and call you when they are about to pass out and say, 'Well, they thought it would stop and it was just diarrhea.' Or they will vomit blood for a few days and not call you until they are hypotensive and can't even walk anymore. When you explain to them that maybe drinking a fifth of vodka a day may have something to do with it, they look at you surprised.

When you're on call for the copter, it's not a lot different. It certainly is an excellent service for the patients because we're the only program in the area that sends an emergency medicine resident onboard to the scene. The others only have nurses or paramedics. They're good, but physicians can make lots of decisions on-site. They can change the standard protocol for handling things without having to waste time checking with home base; sometimes those few minutes make the difference between survival and going down the tube.

But I don't think the copter experience adds much to training. Mostly, you're seeing the same things that you would if you went out in the Bronco. Once in a while, you get into a hostage situation or some people trapped on a mountain road, but these are the exceptions. Usually, you are simply dealing with things at a greater distance, so you need the chopper. Sometimes, it can get you into a very unpleasant situation, especially with interhospital transfers. You often end up in remote hospitals where the ER doc is a retired anesthesiologist. It happened to me recently. There was this older woman who the ER doc told the family, 'Your mother is going to die. She has a malignant cardiac rhythm.' He sent her up to their cardiac unit. The head nurse up there was sharp enough to know she was in V-tach, and she took responsibility for calling us. We found the woman had been shocked some 30 times and had third-degree burns on her chest—but had been given nothing by way of meds. We treated her immediately and flew her back to the hospital. She was discharged well five days later. I hate situations like that. Even if you know what you're doing, it's a professional land mine.

In another hospital, we were called in for an accident case. It was clear right away that the woman had an expanding pneumothorax and needed a chest tube before we could fly her out. The ER doc refused, and I kept insisting because I was afraid of what would happen in the copter if we didn't get the tube in ahead of time. Finally, he took me out in the hall and admitted he didn't know how to put one in, so I told him I'd be glad to do it. We went back into the room, and he started firing off orders to the nurses and to me. I didn't say anything. I just put the tube in, and we flew her back.

A couple of weeks ago, we flew out to this small hospital that had a bad trauma patient they couldn't handle. The doctor met us at the door with the patient on a gurney and wouldn't let us come in. He insisted we load the patient on the copter at once before we even examined her. I didn't fight about it. We just took her out into the parking lot under the lights, examined her, got an airway in, started some blood, immobilized her, and then got her onboard. You have to learn to handle those situations like a UN diplomat. It's not like going to an accident scene, where you're the person in charge and you run things.

These anecdotes bring back lots of memories for me. While I was still a premed student, I spent some time working as an emergency room orderly. As I look back, I realize how much gross negligence there was on the part of the staff, partly because there were no ER-trained physicians there, but also because there was no prehospital care and nobody in the ER had any clear picture of what had happened to the patient—what the scene looked like or what the family was like. Now, we have the ability to be at somebody's house if there's a cardiac arrest in four or five minutes. I'm not talking about just the paramedics, I'm talking about a doctor.

This gives us the capacity to do almost anything in the field that we can do in the ER. We can even bring blood on the copter so that someone who is entrapped out on the turnpike in a semitrailer and is in hypovolemic shock can get three or four units of blood while they're being extricated.

I also enjoy the variety of ERs we work in. There are three different general ERs we rotate through in addition to the specialty hospitals like OB/GYN, psychiatry, and pediatrics. You need to use a different philosophy and approach in each one because the attendings and the residents vary in each. In one place, it's almost like private practice. I call you at 2 A.M. to talk about one of your patients who has walked in, and I admit your patient. There is no dialogue and very little teaching. At the second place, there is more dialogue, but it's not academic. At the University Hospital, there's a lot more protocol about who you call and in what order, but there's much more teaching. I think that's fantastic. It teaches you how to function in any kind of setting.

What I'm telling you is that there's tremendous variation in the attendings you run into. The kind of attending I look for is one who can be your friend and your mentor and yet provide leadership, someone who knows when to push the hell out of you but, at the same time, is sensitive to your needs, who can say to you, 'Hey, it's very slow now, and you've worked all day yesterday and been on all night. Why don't you go home and get some sleep? I'll take care of it here.' You would be amazed how rarely that happens.

Someday, if I'm an attending, I expect to push the residents very hard to achieve. And yet, I hope that when somebody looks like a train wreck and we are not terribly busy, I can send him or her home to get some Zs, and I'll pick up the pieces. Many of the attendings who have seen the program grow, with more and more demands on the residents, still seem somewhat insensitive to the way we are stretched. They don't always step in when we need them. Most of them are young because the field itself is so new, and yet they forget very fast what it's like to be a house officer.

It means a lot to me for somebody to say, 'Joe, you looked bashed in. Go home. We can handle it. It won't be a laundromat tomorrow when you come back.' But believe me, it happens once in a blue moon. It's the same thing in medicine and surgery. I see those interns so abused. That's all it is: abuse. I don't see some senior resident saying to an intern, 'Look, you've just admitted the last 13 patients. Go to bed. I'll do this H and P.' It's kind of like 'I had to do it, so you have to do it.' It's like hazing. You are a plebe at West Point.

The up side of all this is that I am very high on emergency medicine—more than ever. One of the things I like is that you can't get bored either with the knowledge base or the practice—it's infinite. Things like pediatrics or OB or neurosurgery seemed too finite for me. I felt if I did one of those for 10 years, I'd get stale. I would know pretty much what I needed to know and things would start getting routine. In this speciality, what you have to master is boundless, and you are constantly challenged. I read all the time. I'd read the toilet paper if there were any print on it. I just soak up this stuff like a sponge. Everything attracts me. I want to know about the new cardiovascular drugs, about new suture material coming out, about new resuscitation equipment, and so on.

Once in a while, I moonlight at some little bohunk hospital and some kid comes in with pneumonia. I'm there all alone like a doc in a box. So I run home later and read as much as I can get my hands on about pediatric pneumonia. There's no end to the excitement of this.

A lot of people still don't understand what is unique about emergency medicine. That's probably why there were so many turf battles for a while with surgery and medicine. We don't want their cases. We're just a link in the chain. We're the people who can make things right for them to do their thing better.

Let me contrast two recent cases for you to make my point. In one hospital where we work, the residents are kind of lazy. They don't read. They don't work very hard. This patient comes into the ER, in his 50s with mid-abdominal pain and radiation to the back. He was nauseated and vomited. He had weakness in both legs. His blood pressure was 80 over 40, and he had a racing pulse. He had a tender pulsating mass in his belly. Communication was tough because he spoke with a heavy Italian accent. The odds were very high that this was an abdominal aneurysm. I immediately called surgery and told them what was up and that I was afraid he was dissecting. Two and a half hours later, he died in the OR because it took them so long to get to it. And even then, they futzed around forever with a lot of other diagnoses and studies that were unnecessary because they just didn't know what the odds were. I couldn't convince these surgical residents that they shouldn't be treating him for angina or pancreatitis. In the meantime, I was pouring blood lactate solution and wide-open dopamine into this guy, and I couldn't get his pressure up. These people were absolutely refractory. I finally called their attending and said, 'Goddammit! This man has an aneurysm.' They finally scanned him, but he died in the OR a little while later. I was furious. I made sure those residents got their asses burned for that.

Okay. Contrast that with an experience in another hospital where we work. I was sitting in the ER about ten o'clock last Saturday morning having a cup of coffee, and the medics come in and say they have this guy—very strange: some weakness in both legs and some flank pain on one side. His pressure was way down. We got some fluids in him, and his pressure began to come up. He was starting to arrest, and he was in and out of consciousness. Who walks by but the cardiovascular surgeon? I grabbed him, and I said this patient has some rectal tenderness, and I think he has some free blood in his peritoneal cavity. I had already scheduled him for a CT scan. He was in the OR in 30 minutes. He had a large abdominal aneurysm that was dissecting and rupturing. They were able to save him. From the minute he walked into the ER until they had his abdomen open was less than an hour. That made me feel good. That guy didn't slip through the cracks. We never should have lost the other one.

Now, if residents don't respond quickly enough, I'll just go around them. I don't care if they burn. Maybe it's just different philosophies in different hospitals. In some places, if you sound worried, they're there in a couple of minutes. In others, they lumber in 15 minutes later, and they spend so much time arguing with you that the patient can die right under your nose.

It's just a whole different way of looking at patient care. Because you are the first link in the chain, if the rest of the links don't hang together, you're pretty worthless—and you also begin to look incompetent because your patients are dying on you. Now, my way of handling that stress is to call the attending at home and tell him to get his resident down here—and I don't want him getting a bunch of serum amylases and other cardiac studies while this acute appendicitis patient perforates on me. Most attendings are grateful because it reduces their liability and keeps their residents on their toes.

People are getting wise to this stuff. I've talked to employees of hospitals who don't have emergency-medicine trained physicians in their ER. Now I see them sitting in the ER of some hospital where we work. They've had the experience of waiting for hours in acute pain, like from renal colic, on a couple of Tylenols because there's nobody walking around prioritizing care. That's the worst kind of medicine, and you won't find it where ER docs work. They're trained to do triage and organize care. God, how much judgment does it take to say that you want to see a patient with angina before one with a broken leg?!—even if the angina patient comes in second. And then you've got interns sending patients out who shouldn't go out. Even the paramedics come to me and ask why such and such a patient with chest pain was sent home instead of being kept overnight for observation and studies.

Basically, I'm very happy with the training. I wish the leadership of the program would spend more time with us so we could learn more from them. They're the real reason I chose this residency, but we don't have much contact with them. Something should be done about that. Also, if I were the residency training director, I would kick some asses. I would spell out very clearly what the requirements are, and people who didn't meet them would be put on probation. Then, if that didn't pull up their socks, they'd be out. I give 150%, and I want to see some intensity in the people and some commitment or I'd get rid of them. At the same time, I'd try to be a little more sensitive, as I said before: when somebody hasn't had a Friday night off in three weeks, I'd arrange for them to spend some time with their family or get some sleep. I hope I don't forget what I'm saying when I get to be an attending. I really hope I don't.

▲   ▲   ▲

This group of house officers, perhaps more than any other I interviewed, wanted to talk about their cases. A significant portion of every interview was occupied by surprisingly detailed descriptions of clinical encounters on highways; in third–floor–back bedrooms in old, dilapidated homes; in first-aid rooms in football stadiums; on mountainsides; and in isolated farmhouses. They seemed mindful of the drama attendant on their work. Obviously, there are many risks involved in the high-speed rescue attempts and in the helicopter flights, but I heard no complaints or regrets.

They also used their case illustrations skillfully to educate the outsider who might be ignorant about the potential contributions of their specialty. Apparently, they had been involved in many turf battles, particularly with surgery and internal medicine, for control of the emergency room in hospitals. Like many other specialists, they felt little understood and often unappreciated. Dr. W. explained his position very neatly as he talked about his contribution being "one link in the chain" of care for an acutely ill patient—of his ability to do things in emergency situations based on his training that would make it easier for the surgeon or the internist to be effective at later stages of the game. But with regret, many of these people talked about their colleagues being threatened by the presence of emergency medicine attendings and house officers in the environs. They often perceived themselves as being engaged in a battle for the possession of the patient rather than fitting into a continuum of care.

The concomitant pride that was felt in being able to do something very special, something that even many of the medical seniors would not know how to do, shone through in much of the discussion about patients. In describing one of his early experiences, a second-year house officer said:

▼   ▼   ▼

I was on copter call. We were notified at 3 A.M. about a motorcycle accident way out in the boondocks. Apparently, the guy was drunk, wearing no helmet, and hit the side of a barn at high speed on his cycle. He was taken to a local hospital where the emergency room was staffed by an experienced surgeon, but somebody who had not had any training in emergency medicine. They really couldn't deal with this patient. While I was in transit in the copter, we got a report that he had head and chest injuries and a tense abdomen. The only thing that had been done for him was that he had been immobilized on a board. At that point, I had been out of my internship one month. In flight, I was changing my underwear and getting dressed while the information was coming in on the radio. The attending at the hospital was very senior to me, but here he was calling me for help. My own attending was 100 miles away. I could talk to him on the phone if I wanted to, but all he would say was that it was my judgment. By the time we got there, the patient was struggling and irrational. I intubated him, I got in some large lines and fluid going, and I paralyzed him in order to stop his thrashing around. I did all this before we even took off. He did well, and I felt very good about it.

That was the first time I was in a major situation by myself with no help. The whole thing was up to me. I knew what to do, but before there had always been somebody above me to say 'You're right. Go ahead and do it.' This guy weighed 250 pounds and was rolling around on the gurney. How was I going to intubate him without paralyzing him? It was very scary but it came out all right.

▲   ▲   ▲

The above case illustrates very nicely what is so attractive to young people about this specialty. It certainly appeals to one's rescue fantasies. My impression, also, is that another appeal has to do with the short-term involvement with patients, the rapid turnover, the quick results (whether good or bad), and the feeling of "anything goes" because there are no boundaries to the specialty. One must immediately do what is needed on the scene. The constant stretching of one's knowledge and capacities is stimulating and enjoyable. Dr. W., from whom we have already heard, seemed very pleased with what he described as the "infinite" knowledge base in this specialty. He described how he might become bored doing other kinds of medical work because they were "finite." He said, "In this specialty, what you have to master is boundless, and you are constantly challenged."

Dr. V. who was a 27-year-old second-year resident, said about emergency medicine, "This is not a field for people who like a lot of follow-up on their patients and who need to see long-range outcome. Most of it is one-shot deals, and you have to hope for quick results or at least the knowledge that you have stabilized the patient and that she or he is ready for the next step in the treatment process. There is very little feedback unless you go chasing after all the patients, and you don't have time for that—maybe just an occasional one that interests you especially. If you find that kind of life frustrating, this is the wrong business for you. And the other thing is that you have to be able to take criticism well because everything you do is in a fishbowl."

The "boundless" nature of the specialty turns out to be something of a two-edged sword. In this program, there are, indeed, almost an unlimited number of opportunities to use the emergency medicine house officers. Although some found this challenging and exciting, they were all beginning to find that they were being stretched too thin and feared burnout. Dr. W. said of the training:

▼   ▼   ▼

Mostly, it's what I wanted, and although there is some stress in being out in the field on your own, that is really why I went into this training in the first place. The kind of stresses you find in this residency that ought to be fixed have to do with the fact that we are getting too stretched. For instance, we have to cover all the NFL games in this area, and the marathon, and most of the big university football games. We also cover all the big events in town, like rock concerts and parades. All of this is in addition to the emergency room and radio call and the chopper and trying to get some research done, too—I forgot that we also have to teach all the advanced-cardiac-life-support courses and also the basic courses, and we do a lot of formal training of the paramedics, and we give a lot of talks to outside groups. I think we need to look at our priorities and reorganize them. We either need to give up some of these peripheral things or enlarge the residency to include more people. There is too much effort to please too many people. It's funny, but we only have to send two guys to the NFL games but four to the college games. I guess they think the kids are going to be more violent and that there will be more drunkenness at the college games, and they are probably right!

▲   ▲   ▲

The responsibility of working with the paramedics was seen as both stressful and desirable by these house officers. They seemed to understand that emergency medicine programs that are focused strictly within a hospital and provide no pre-hospital training are deficient. They understood that the opportunity that this program provided to have extensive field experience with patients before they were actually admitted to the hospital was crucial.

Dr. W. said, "Being able to go out into the field and see a side of medicine nobody else ever sees trains you in ways that you can't even approach in the hospital. You need to learn how to work with many different people. We have 160 paramedics, and in the end, you need to work with all of them. You are constantly adapting to their styles and their level of experience. You have to learn to work in incredible environments. You encounter patients the way they are in their setting, and you have to decide on the spot what to do with them. If you can do that, you can handle anything in a hospital. I feel so much more comfortable with whatever rolls into the hospital door now, after the experience in the field, where it is so much tougher to work. I think better in the hospital now because I have gone through so much worse on the outside. In addition, it gives you better insight into what the patient has gone through. You see on the hoof what people can do to other people, the violence, the destructiveness, and what they can do to themselves in car accidents and suicides."

At the same time, the one-shot nature of the clinical exposure that they gave to patients left them bereft of any sense of continuity with the patient as a member of a family system, a workplace, a career, or a social being. In contrast to the family practice residents, from whom we will hear shortly, the exposure of these trainees to the patient's life was like a microtome slice. They were not unaware of this. One resident said, "Most cardiac arrests are now run in the field. There is the family standing behind you as you work, and then the paramedics take the patient to the hospital, and the family is left behind in a state of shock and there is no one around to pick up the pieces or help them. Many of the patients don't survive, and sometimes it has been a very messy arrest with trauma, people falling down the steps, and the family is left to clean everything afterward with no help. There is no provision made for anyone to go in and really help the family through that transition. We can't do it because we have to stay with the patient, but you can only imagine what is going on as the patient is suddenly yanked from his or her normal setting within a few minutes. It opens your eyes in a way you never thought of before. When a patient rolls into the ER without that, all you see is this patient in cardiac arrest. You don't know anything else. I'm sorry that we can't help the families, but it's not our job to do that. Our job is to stay with the patient and try to save him."

The helicopter has added an interesting dimension to their experience. Most felt that the helicopter was not essential in terms of their training, but that it probably did give access to some patients who were either not accessible by car or not reachable soon enough. One resident said,

▼   ▼   ▼

About half the copter flights you go on really aren't necessary as copter flights, but it is hard to tell ahead of time. Sometimes, having the doctor there instead of just nurses or paramedics means that you can make a decision that they can't. They have to go by the book, there is a drill they have to follow, but you can make a decision to individualize care in a different way. Some of the flights involve transfer from hospital to hospital, and you learn a lot from going to outlying hospitals on trauma cases about what hasn't been done that is sometimes very obvious. You pick up patients that have not had the right procedures or studies done on them, and the big problem is to get them back to the medical center as fast as possible so they can get to the OR, where immediate intervention is possible. How you handle this with the attendings and the nurses at the outlying hospitals is very tricky because you don't want to look like a smartass. Sometimes you are dealing with an attending who is 30 years your senior. You are going to a hospital where the patient has been for several hours, and you expect certain things to have been done and they are not. It's almost like going to a home or a highway accident. If you know how to be diplomatic, you can teach at the same time, and that's very satisfying.

Sometimes, you are in a situation with experienced flight nurses and paramedics where they have many years of experience and you have to put yourself in the position to learn from them and yet still be the physician in charge, and that takes some fancy footwork. You get to feeling that you should be a whole lot smarter than you are. You have to set up a trade-off situation. They can teach us more how to handle a jumper or an extrication from a car, but we can teach them, maybe, what to do for that man during the 20 minutes that he's being freed from the car because we have a hunch that maybe we could predict from looking at the car what kind of hidden damage there may be or how to administer specialized care to the patient while all of this is going on. You just have to prevent yourself from getting defensive and to remember that you're part of a team. If you listen to a scanner and listen to all the medic channels in the city, you would hear a lot of back and forth between the paramedics and the docs, with the docs giving instructions but the medics making suggestions and asking questions. Very often, the doc will say, 'Do you need anything else or do you have any other ideas?' and they will come up with things.

It takes a lot more sophistication than I ever dreamed. You are dealing with several hospitals, several specialties, attendings and residents and out-lying hospitals, flight nurses, and paramedics who often know more than you do about a specific thing, so you are always picking your way through this diplomatic mine field. Sure, there is a lot of content to learn, but the con-tent is worthless unless you learn how to deal with systems and vice versa.

Sometimes you see our residents sitting at a desk just thoroughly pooped or spaced out, and you have the feeling that you just want to go away for a month. We are always on trial because we are so young as a specialty and are being pulled in so many different directions. I think about the saying that a woman has to be twice as good at her job as a man to be recognized. I think we are in that position as a specialty.

▲   ▲   ▲

Although the attendings were generally liked and respected, the system for monitoring radio calls was found to be very stressful by most younger residents. Dr. V. stated, "There is always an attending listening on exactly the same radio as you've got, so if he doesn't like what you're telling the paramedics, he can jump in and change things. There is always an attending looking over your shoulder when you are on the radio, and that is extremely stressful, especially in the second year, when you are not all that sure of yourself yet."

Dr. S., a 30-year-old senior resident seemed to have a bit more perspective and felt that things were changing for his specialty. He said, "In some of the emergency rooms where we work, medicine and surgery residents are likely to turn to us as consultants because this is a small part of their work and we do very little else, so they often use us to learn the fastest way to handle acute situations as they come in. Left to their own devices, they are likely to do things in the ER that they learned in medical school, and many of them went to school where there were no ER-trained attendings, so they just learned from internists and surgeons. That's why emergency medicine is so hard to pigeon-hole. It's something of everything; it's both a medical and a surgical specialty. At first, surgeons and internists were a lot more threatened by us than they are now. I believe there is less of a turf battle than used to be true. We don't want to take their patients out of the OR, but we can teach their residents how to do an emergency assessment on an acute surgical patient a lot faster and easier. Maybe they are beginning to relax more now, even in other specialties. There aren't too many 50-year-old ENT people who want to come in at 3 A.M. to see an acute otitis media patient of theirs, especially if they know you can handle it very well until they are in in the morning."

So, here we see a group of house officers largely enjoying what they were doing but fearing burnout because they were constantly being pulled in many directions and were asked to be available to carry our multiple functions. At the same time, they had to learn to work in an extremely complex health-care-delivery system and with attendings and paraprofessionals who might not always understand or appreciate the contribution they could make.

Chapter 17

Family Practice

Dr. O. is a 28-year-old second-year resident in family practice. His wife is a nurse and is employed by the Visiting Nurse Society. They have a five-month-old infant daughter. He was originally from a small New England town, where he went to school and where he plans to open a practice on completion of this residency. He is a very big man, perhaps 6′ 5″ in height and 230 pounds in weight. He is balding, and the thin, silky wisps of his remaining hair hang over his forehead like a fringe. The sleeves of his dark tartan shirt were rolled above his elbows. Poking from his shirt pocket were three dark cheroots, which, thankfully, remained there for the duration of the interview. He sat down on the sofa in my office and propped his size 14Es on the coffee table, signaling the degree of comfort he felt in talking with me.

▼   ▼   ▼

I knew what I wanted to do from the time I was in high school. I was interested in a general medical practice in a small town, and I've never had any second thoughts about it. Any conflict I've experienced has come during the residency in dealing with other specialists, particularly those who may feel a little threatened by my specialty. Maybe they're feeling a bit crowded by us—like Pediatrics and OB/GYN and perhaps internal medicine. There's some hostility there, which I guess is unavoidable. Even during training, I run into some of this among other residents or attendings. In all honesty, I guess it's kind of two-sided. There's some insecurity in our group about whether we really know enough in all these areas to do a good job.

You can't help feeling a little insecure sometimes. But as I go along, I feel better about myself. I know that, sometimes, I'm projecting my insecurity in various situations, and I get a little paranoid. The attitude we seem to be running into a lot in these other specialists is that they believe we're doing the same things that they are—we're just not doing them as well!

When I was a med student, my school had a family practice residency, and I heard the other residents putting them down out of earshot—that they were not of the same quality or didn't know as much. They made a big issue of how hard they were working on the wards while the family practice residents were working in the office lollygagging around with patients who weren't all that sick anyway and anybody could do that kind of work.

Maybe we've gotten something of an image among the residents who have to do a lot more inpatient work than we do, that this is sort of a cushy residency. It isn't. We have to cover so much material, and we have to be constantly adjusting to new settings. That puts a lot of stress and strain on your nervous system. For instance, this second year is divided into 10 five-week rotations. It includes pediatrics, OB/GYN, internal medicine, emergency room, the intensive care unit, psychiatry, and a few electives.

This has its good and bad aspects. The good part is that you get tremendous exposure to different patient populations and different attendings. It's a broad experience. The bad part is that you are constantly moving around the city to a variety of hospitals, which means always having to learn new procedures, new rules, new forms and paperwork, and new head nurses who have their own little idiosyncrasies. What helps is that this is maybe the third or fourth time around. You sort of do this in medical school in your third-year clinical clerkships and, to some degree, in your fourth year and then again as an intern, so you get a bit accustomed to this constant changing, and each time your chain feels yanked a little less. Also, each time you come back to a particular specialty, you don't start from scratch. You learn a little more, so you get more expertise in each area.

The first priority for me when I get to a new hospital is to figure out what has to be done and how to get it done efficiently. I'm not too concerned with going to teaching conferences or lectures or that kind of stuff. You can always get to that later, once you've got a handle on things. Anyway, you learn the most from your patients and your attendings, and that's what you retain over time. I tend to go to very few teaching conferences. I was a student for over 20 years, and I need to learn in other ways now.

I'm likely to spend a fair amount of time getting friendly and sidling up to the nurses and the ward secretaries in a new setting, so they will teach me the system quickly; social skills with those people are crucial. You have to learn how to kibitz with them. I try to learn how to get things done with a minimum of hassles and without wasting a lot of time. I hate to fumble around. It's these people who can help you early on even more than the attendings, who have more technical information, much of which you already know anyway.

In most hospitals, we can function fairly independently because we are now licensed physicians. You check with the attending, especially if you're not sure of something. In our home-based hospital, we're usually the senior physician present and are pretty much on our own except when we ask for help. The only place where they treat us any differently is the Children's Hospital, where we serve as pediatric interns. I didn't enjoy being an intern again after having all this responsibility. They feel we don't know enough pediatrics to function as residents, but let me tell you that, in many ways, we're ahead of where their residents are in knowing how to get information from families, how to use the family in developing the treatment plan, and how to use the right community resources for a child who has a chronic, disabling illness. They could learn a lot from us, but they don't.

The Children's Hospital experience was very unpleasant for this reason. It's very upsetting to be forced into a position where you have no responsibility and are treated like a rank beginner. It's hard to justify all that misery for what you learn there. It isn't that you don't learn; you do. But I wonder if we couldn't learn it under other circumstances.

No matter what hospital we're currently assigned to, we have to round first thing in the morning at our own hospital on any inpatients we have had to admit from the clinics we run. We also have two different sets of office hours per week in our continuity clinic for the patients we follow. For me, this is the best part of the week because these are the patients I really get to know. You see everything from acute infections, vaginitis, pelvic inflammatory disease, and other gynecology to long-term chronic things like hypertension, diabetes, and so on. The other thing I like about it is that you are doing everything from well-baby care to geriatrics. How can you get bored?

Even though most of the practice of medicine is ambulatory care, in most residencies they emphasize inpatient care and sort of use the clinics as an add-on. I don't think that's very good training. In our residency, the emphasis is on ambulatory care, even though you spend a fair amount of time on the floors; the basic understanding is that practice mostly involves taking care of patients outside the hospital, and that's what they prepare you for.

But in or out of the hospital, the patient is yours: if they get pregnant, we take care of them; if they get a heart attack, we take care of them. We can get expert consultation from various specialties if necessary, but we don't let go of the patients regardless of what happens to them.

This is what brought me into this specialty, and it's where the major satisfactions come from. If you were to ask about a case I found especially rewarding, here's a good example. Actually, it involves an elderly married couple in their 80s. Initially, the wife was the patient. She was a long-term diabetic with lots of trouble being stabilized. She had bad leg and foot ulcers. She was very obese and had multiple complaints. She didn't take good care of herself. I would say she had kind of a passive–aggressive personality. She was a whiner. They always came in as a pair. The husband would talk about his wife's problems but never about himself very much.

At one point, he started to complain of abdominal pain. When I examined him, he had what appeared to be an inguinal hernia but what turned out to be a mass that was filled with metastatic carcinoma. We never did find out where the primary site was. We started him on regular chemotherapy, which I administered to him as an outpatient after much discussion back and forth with him and other family members about the risks and benefits. It involved my being able to give enormous support to them on multiple visits. I even discussed with the family what to do if he should stop breathing—which did happen while I was at another hospital.

I worked with the wife and the daughter afterward. I helped with the grief reaction. I even helped with all the paperwork surrounding his death and burial because they were so confused and upset by everything. I continued to work with the wife after he died. Recently, she couldn't manage by herself anymore, so she moved to the South to live with her daughter. That whole experience was very satisfying for me. At first, it was stressful to deal with all those things at once—all the treatments, the family counseling, the death, all the complications—but I learned to do it, and the family was very grateful to me for the way I managed the case. See, for me, that was a success despite the inevitable outcome. I feel I gave the best possible care.

Incidentally, my psychiatric rotation is coming up in a few months, and I'm going to request to spend the whole five weeks on geriatrics. It's the kind of situation I just described that makes me think that's the best way to use the time. I'm not going to be taking care of schizophrenics or infantile autism, but I will be running into lots of aged patients who are decompensating. You have to know the difference between some organic brain disorder and depression and that kind of stuff so you know what to do with them and what to tell the families. I'm very ignorant in that area now.

Medical training doesn't prepare you very well to work with families. You never know enough about this. Most doctors don't even try very hard. Where you see good examples of this is in the ICU. You can have a patient who was at home with a terminal malignancy. They suddenly go into cardiac arrest and are brought in by the paramedics. You don't know what's going on. The family wants you to keep this hopeless patient alive on some life-support system. He may be already brain-dead, and you are faced with an enormous amount of work trying to keep somebody alive where there is little or no point to it. You are not doing anything for the patient. You are not learning anything. You are just satisfying the guilt of some family member who may have just flown in from out of town and hasn't seen the patient in years. Often, it's just one family member, and the rest of the family is against what you are doing, but you have to satisfy that one person because they are so adamant.

Usually, this is the result of the attending's not having spent enough time with the family previously to let them know what the realities are and what the options are. He or she hasn't explained the total situation to them. We had this woman brought into the ICU recently who had a bilateral mastectomy. She had an indwelling catheter for chemotherapy. I learned that she had been going to a pain center for nine weeks and just wanted to die. The internist had never discussed this with the family. We had no idea what was going on. I resuscitated her, but nobody wanted me to. The internist had never communicated with us either. In the end, she didn't live very long, but that is bad medical practice. When I told the internist we had started her heart again, he said, 'Great job. Nice going.' I was thinking, 'Where are you? What planet are you from?' I felt terrible when he congratulated me. It was the first compliment I ever had that upset me.

So sometimes you are stuck with all this fruitless work and this very bad situation in the ICU. It's a symptom of poor medical practice as far as I'm concerned. It means poor communication—or total lack of it. It's no wonder there are so many malpractice suits.

Residents have a pretty clear idea who the good attendings are very quickly. First, you want somebody who gives a damn about teaching and who makes some investment in it, who isn't always looking at his or her watch in a hurry to get back to the office. That means trusting you to take care of his or her patients but keeping an eye on what you're doing and interacting with you so you learn without the feeling you're being spoon-fed. They have to be able to delegate responsibility and not argue with you over every little point if they don't agree 100% with what you're doing.

They also role-model more than they think they do because you see them sending patients in, and you know how they practice and what they have told people. It involves not only how they handle people medically, but some of the social and interpersonal aspects of practice. As I said before, how they handle the family—issues around death and dying. I'm impressed by attendings who can stay on top of things, keep the family in the picture, and develop a good treatment contract with the patient, who understand what the patients want out of treatment and out of their life, and how they feel about termination of treatment if it should be necessary—somebody who doesn't practice by the numbers but individualizes every case.

I watch how they make decisions about hospitalizing a patient: which patients really need hospitalization and which ones don't. Are they dumping the patient in the hospital because they don't have the persistence or the interest to really work the patient up carefully in the office and they want us to do the work for them? Or are they dumping the patient in the hospital for economic reasons because they will be reimbursed more if they round quickly on inpatients every day? You can tell, and these things make a difference.

You learn from both the positive and the negative. Either way, you begin to develop some very strong ideas about the kind of doctor you want to be—and the kind you don't want to be.

▲   ▲   ▲

It should be evident, even to the casual observer, that the typical house officers' training in the family practice field had some things in common with their counterparts in emergency medicine but, in many ways are different critters. Although they want to avoid specializing, are interested in patients of all ages, and have a curiosity about all diseases and their treatment, it appears that they receive their most important professional rewards in quite different ways. They want a broader, longer-lasting involvement with the patient and the family and are willing to settle for partial goals to delay gratification for considerable periods of time in order to gain a sense of success. I can't escape the impression that these two groups are the heads and tails of the same coin.

Dr. F., who was a 27-year-old second-year resident in family practice, described his own value system and used a pointed case illustration this way:

▼   ▼   ▼

What I'm learning, in general, is that practice is made up of a lot of these minor little triumphs—on a good day. There aren't any dramatic successes. Those, you read about in *Time*. My own continuity clinic consists of a lot of people I'm just trying to keep out of the hospital. That is a big problem with many of them. They have such complex lives and so many frustrating things wrong that you can't fix.

One of the most difficult patients I have to deal with is a 22-year-old black woman who has repeated episodes of thrombosis of the deep veins in all four extremities. We can't figure out why. She doesn't use drugs: she has no needle tracks, and her urine drug screens are always negative. It's been something of a success just establishing a relationship with her because she has been very noncompliant in the past with other doctors and very irresponsible. In the year before I met her, she was in the hospital three or four times to remove the clots surgically. In the year and a half since I've known her, she's only had to have one hospitalization because she's keeping her clinic appointments and taking her Coumadin.

I guess the difference is that I've been there for her—met with her frequently, kept after her, and been available for every little question and phone call she has. I've kept encouraging her. Now she calls frequently about very little things even when she doesn't really need me, but I take the calls anyway. She just seems to need the contact with me. It's like if I'm willing to put the effort in, then she's willing to, also. In spite of the fact that she's a load, she's a patient I can do something for, and there are good results, so it's worth it.

▲   ▲   ▲

This sense of triumph, limited though it may seem, achieved through simply keeping a patient stable and out of the hospital with admittedly modest gains was very typical of the thinking of these house officers. This sense of long-term involvement in a patient's care regardless of the ups and downs of life provided a sense of contributing in a more substantial way than what one resident described as a "hit-or-miss" kind of practice. Dr. O., from whom we heard at the beginning of this chapter, described at length his feeling of reward from working with an elderly couple for long periods of time when he knew complete recovery was out of the question.

Dr. N., another second-year resident talked about his orientation this way:

▼   ▼   ▼

The fun of medicine is the people, the patients. That's why I like the work in the family health center. I've gotten involved not only in their medical problems but in their total life situations.

One lady I'm following right now has rheumatic heart disease. She's in her late 50s. Her educational level and her ability to articulate about what is happening to her body are extremely limited. Sometimes, I feel almost like I'm practicing veterinary medicine with her. I first saw her about a year and a half ago when she came in complaining of dizziness. Now she comes in and will show me her new pair of tennis shoes. She had been worked up at another hospital very extensively, and they hadn't been able to find any cause for her dizziness.

I continued to study her and watch her closely and picked up some atrial fibrillation at a very slow rate. I put her in the hospital and got her stabilized on the right medication. Her dizziness went down considerably. She has since been in and out of the hospital several times, with the dizziness increasing and decreasing. A lot of it depends on how compliant she is with her medication, but I've learned a lot of other things about her as we talk. She's involved in a bad custody case for her granddaughter against her own daughter. She raised the granddaughter, and now the daughter wants her back—it's been extremely stressful for her. So, I've gotten involved in the whole family scene, trying to help them work this out. There are still many times when she claims dizziness when there's no clear reason for it. Often, all examinations and lab studies are normal.

Once, it turned out there was a hearing before a judge concerning the child, and the hearing had to be canceled because she was in the hospital with one of her dizzy spells. As soon as it was canceled, she started to feel better and wanted to be discharged. I feel her heart is not the whole reason for her physical complaints. I have tried to get into this other business with her, with very modest results, but I have another year in the program, and it is a challenge.

▲   ▲   ▲

One can only be grateful that doctors are as different and come in as many varieties as do their patients! As I listened to these family practice residents, I experienced a sense of gratitude and relief to know that there are some physicians who can experience gratification working with their patients in a world of high technology and cravings for instant satisfaction. This, in no way, diminished my respect and admiration for and thankfulness about all of the bright quick residents in the surgical specialties.

What about the stresses faced by this group of house officers? Dr. O. who opened this chapter, spoke eloquently about the problems of having to circulate through so many systems and relate to so many different individuals. He also described how he coped with this by ingratiating himself with the nursing staffs in each setting. He also said about the breadth of his specialty that it was, in some ways, limitless because it cut across all other specialties.

Dr. N. agreed and had these cogent comments to make: "In college, I was involved with a very scholarly faculty member, and I learned something from that exposure that will stick with me, that is, self-teaching skills. A fair amount of self-teaching is part of all residencies, but nobody helps you with how to do that and how to maintain it after you're out on your own, which is why so many doctors become hacks. Once they're out of the residency, where there are always attendings around to help them with something new, they don't know how to stay on top of new knowledge as it comes out and how to apply it to their practice. I think I could tell you now which people in our program are not going to do well on their own."

As was the case with the emergency medicine house officers, there was this sense of not being understood or appreciated by other specialties, a feeling of mutual threat. As Dr. O. said, "The attitude we seem to be running into a lot in these other specialists is that they believe we're doing the same things they are—we're just not doing them as well!" Sometimes, there was even a sense of being rather persecuted because, as they rotated from hospital to hospital, they saw themselves assigned the menial role of intern rather than resident and felt they were again being unappreciated. Every house officer whom I interviewed in this specialty expressed this concern about being deprecated by other specialists.

One who had entered training bright-eyed and bushy-tailed and expecting to enjoy himself in a lifetime of immersing himself in the health care of families said that he was often discouraged by the experience because he felt he did not always have the know-how or the tools to help many of the people who came to him. He said,

▼   ▼   ▼

There are lots and lots of patients whom I feel I can't do anything for. When I see their names on my schedule, I say, 'Oh no, not that one again.' All I can do is sit there and listen to their troubles. Most of what is wrong with them is their life, and I can't do anything about that. They're sort of depressed but not enough for a psychiatric referral. They have an alcoholic husband or something. We are all taught to fix things in medical school, and when you have no way to fix something, it's very frustrating.

These experiences are causing me to rethink what I want to do when I finish. I told you my original choice was based on wanting to have long-term contact with families and to give comprehensive care. I didn't want to go into internal medicine because I watched those residents and didn't like them. They were too much like nerds—very rigid and compulsive and very harried. The family practice residents seemed more comfortable and more happy. But my mind is shifting on some of this. I'm finding out some things about myself in the process. I'm not enjoying the experiences as much as I thought I would. It's not the patients so much; it's me. These long-term relationships with patients are not so terribly rewarding.

▲   ▲   ▲

On balance, however, despite the pressures, the stresses, the sense of not always being an equal among equals, most of the group appeared satisfied and on course. After complaining about the pressures he had experienced in trying to deal with so many family problems, Dr. N. said, "Don't misunderstand me. No complaints about the residency. I chose this field because I wanted to be a real doctor—to know what it was like to take care of very sick people while, at the same time, getting a broad experience with different diseases—and I'm getting just that. I'm not sure I want to stay with this as a lifetime career, but whatever I end up doing in medicine, I'll have this under my belt. This experience will keep me from developing a narrow bias, and most specialists have one whether they admit it or not."

So, here we have a group who, in a sense, is working very hard to replace the old-style family doctor, with the awareness that there is now a much larger body of knowledge to master, many more skills to develop, and a surprising degree of unacceptance among one's increasingly super-specialized peers.

BIBLIOGRAPHY

The papers by Nelson, Mazie, and Rudner seem to be consistent with each other and reinforce much of what we have already learned about the balance between stress factors, supports, and coping mechanisms in other specialties. The paper by Parker and Rodney describes an interesting study in which traits of self-discipline were compared with impulsiveness in family practice residents who remained in training versus those who did not after the first year. The study by Rafferty, *et al.* is a well-controlled effort to use a personality inventory to study burnout factors and makes for informative reading.

Nelson EG: Psychosocial factors seen as problems by family practice residents and their spouses. Journal of Family Practice 6:581–589, 1978

Mazie B: Job stress, psychological health, and social support of family practice residents. Journal of Medical Education 60:935–941, 1985.

Rudner HL: Stress and coping mechanisms in a group of family practice residents. Journal of Medical Education 60:564–566, 1985.

Parker J, Rodney WM: Temperament and stress factors predictive of choosing to leave after one year of residency. Family Medicine 18:308–310, 1986.

Rafferty JP, Lemkau JP, Purdy RR, *et al.*: Validity of the Maslach Burnout Inventory for family practice physicians. Journal of Clinical Psychology 42:488–492, 1986.

Part V

GENERIC ISSUES

In the first chapter of this book, I indicated that the plan was to present a word picture of the house officers' experiences in the 16 primary specialties covered. In the next chapters, we looked more at what is specific to each of those specialties than at what is "generic" to postgraduate medical education as revealed by these young physicians.

Now, our immediate task is to do just that. Let me first refer you to Chapter 20, where many of the studies covering these stress areas have been referred to. By *generic stresses*, we mean such problems as fatigue and sleep deprivation, major financial burdens, marital and family tensions, and the incursions into social life and the pursuit of satisfactions outside work that become so difficult during postgraduate training. Other areas we review in that section relate to concerns over the content of training and its usefulness in preparation for future work; problems in the amount and quality of attention given by the attending physicians; and long-range concerns involved in career planning in a profession that is changing very rapidly.

Conceptually, it seems to make greater sense to me not to consider these stresses one by one as part of some long and unrelated laundry list. Rather, they seem to fall into one of two broad, though overlapping, groups: (1) interpersonal and developmental issues and (2) environmental stresses. The two chapters that follow consider these two major areas sequentially. It is important always to remember that, although we are not succumbing to the laundry-list approach, even these major categories interact with and influence each other for better or worse in the daily life of the house officer.

Chapter 18

INTERPERSONAL AND DEVELOPMENTAL ISSUES

It must be obvious that many stresses were identified in the interviews presented so far that have received little attention despite their constant reappearance. It is for this very reason that little effort has been made to discuss them until now. To attempt to do so in our consideration of the various specialties would have been mind-numbing because of the inevitable repetition that would have been required in each chapter. More pointedly, their constant reappearance makes us aware that they must be generic stresses and problems encountered in postgraduate medical education rather than being associated with specific specialties. Some of these problems are "systemic" and are largely determined by environmental conditions that the house officer faces each day in the hospital. We will look at these in the next chapter.

The less obvious but often more troublesome stresses do not involve time, schedules, energy, and the physical environment. They have to do with people: what goes on inside of them and between them. We must also remind ourselves that these house officers themselves are growing and developing human beings, most of them living through an epoch in their own existences that, for most other young people, are very trying times. The transition from late adolescence to productive young adulthood tends to place even stable individuals under stress. For the house officer, that stress is variously reported as a "cold bath" or "baptism of fire." Hence, the title of this chapter.

It is not possible to understand fully the impact of the stresses that are being experienced by these house officers unless they are placed in a developmental context. The age-related struggles for the achievement of a clear identity; the dilemmas associated with becoming a productive worker; the conflicts surrounding the pursuit of intimacy without loss of personal boundaries; the odyssey through dependence, rebellion against authority, and eventual comfort with interdependence; and the achievement of an ego-compatible adult partnership role—all combine to make the decade from the late teens to the late 20s an uncertain and anxiety-filled time for most.

Superimposed on these "normal" developmental tasks are the personal and professional tribulations that our young physicians have already in part described to us.

Let us look at some of the generic problems to which we have paid little attention so far.

TRANSITION FROM STUDENT TO PHYSICIAN

The typical first-year house officer is in the middle 20s and has been primarily a student for 20 years! Although guidance, supervision, and support are usually available, there is no taking away from the fact that this young person is suddenly expected by society—in frog-to-prince like fashion, on July 1 at midnight—to become a physician. Many of our house officers described this as a frightening experience, although almost all described their emotions as being interlaced with feelings of elation and release after so many years of studenthood. The intern confronted with a sudden cardiac arrest at 2 A.M. has no opportunity to call for expert attending physicians to pitch in immediately. These are certainly available soon after the crisis, but emergency decisions and actions are necessary if life is to be preserved. It is this awareness of the inexorable demand created by the patient's illness that, for most house officers, represents their first experience in life with bedrock "reality."

For almost all, given reasonable time and support, this natural dependence of patients provides a maturational stimulus. But the "cold bath" of sudden physicianhood is a state from which it is impossible to protect the house officer.

It not only has an annealing effect on the house officers' internalized picture of themselves as physicians, it appears to be an important determinant of their future choice of specialty. Some interns seem to thrive on crisis situations and on the diagnosis and treatment of patients with very grave disorders. Others seem to eschew the investment necessary to pursue a lifelong career with such patients and move in the direction of specialties with less intense patient contact.

For instance, contrast these two attitudes. First, recall the comments of one of the general surgical house officers, who said, "I like accepting responsibility, making rapid decisions, doing procedures, and seeing quick results. I like the level of authority that's involved. I tried internal medicine for a while, but that's not me. I can't think the way those people do and I can't identify with the personalities in that field." Compare this orientation with that of a radiology resident who said, "I don't mind working hard. I think I'm in the right field. But medicine is not all there is in life. There is something about being able to walk away from the office at night and know that the patients really belong to somebody else and that you have freedom to do other things. There is something about being tied to very sick patients day and night that doesn't fit what I want to do with my life."

It is interesting that some house officers enjoyed their rotations through university-based hospitals more, and that others thrived in community hospitals. Part of the reason seems to be connected with a wish for more involvement with senior physicians and residents, more support and teaching, and more supervision on the part of the first group; and more satisfaction through functioning semiautonomously and "letting the patient be the teacher" on the part of the latter group.

This is a function of different learning styles, and, I believe, evidence that there is more than one road to physicianhood. Some accomplish it best through daily identification with mentors. Others seem to arrive there more easily by spending a period of time immersing themselves in clinical work and learning through direct patient care.

Sadly, still others seem to achieve the role only imperfectly. Many patients can identify these learning failures within the first 15 minutes of encountering their new physician.

THE DYING OR CHRONICALLY IMPAIRED PATIENT

In Chapter 22, there is a series of references describing the stress for new physicians attendant on assuming the responsibility for a dying or severely damaged patient. These should be helpful in arriving at a deeper understanding of this experience. Many trainees report that, although this is always a tribulation, the experience is worst when the patient is a child. For this reason, some house officers, although they enjoy children, stated that they could not endure the pediatric side of their specialty's practice as a career.

A good example of this reaction, you may recall, was expressed by Dr. B., one of the neurology residents, who said, "I could never do pediatric neurology as a career. I would get dragged down very quickly by some of these devastated little kids you see. If you like kids and have your own or are in the process of having them, it can be very scary looking at some of these patients. Before I had my own, it was different. Now I think, 'There but for the grace of God go I.' There's no guarantee. When you by a car, they give you a guarantee, but there's none with a child. It always sticks on me."

And of course, the pediatric house officer himself or herself must face this on almost a daily basis. You will remember Dr. McD., who described his slow adjustment to the reality of death and dying in children this way: "A lot of your initial verve and idealism is stripped away because you know what is coming with a lot of these kids. You've been through it several times, and you know there is no magic. Part of the stress is that you work so hard with these kids trying to save them and they go through so much, and then you end up with the result that you could have had in the first place without all your work and all their agony. You really wonder about it. When death finally happens, it's almost a relief. Sometimes it's the ones who survive that are even worse tragedies because you know what kind of life they and their families have ahead of them."

Although most could not conceptualize it in these terms, what they seemed to be saying was that they had trouble maintaining proper distance from the patient and the family. They found themselves getting too close or too distant. The price for becoming too close is an identification with the patient and, subsequently, a grief reaction that is too much to bear when it occurs repeatedly. The price for emotional distancing is uninvolvement, lack of satisfaction from patient contact, and, ultimately, inappropriate patient care.

For others, there may exist unrealistic motivations for entering medicine. These are threatened when the supposed omnipotence of the physician proves to be a myth, and the patient does not get well—or worse yet, is lost.

Neurosurgical house officers seem to arrive at this identity crisis rather early in their training. They must if they are to survive. Apparently, many enter the field with the so-called Ben Casey identification, an idealized self-image that must be yielded quickly in the face of the incontrovertible evidence that Dr. Casey lives only in the minds of television writers.

Nevertheless, the combined assault of patients who don't get well and diseases about which we know too little represents an enormous stress during the first year of postgraduate training.

Somehow, it is not truly confronted in medical school. It is not until one becomes a physician that a haunting awareness of the limitations of knowledge and skill become day-and-night companions.

MASTERY AND CONTROL ISSUES

Although generally related to the two subjects we have already discussed in this chapter, there is also a whole set of interpersonal parameters that take on additional dimensions. These may not always have to do with death and dying and with the limitations of our knowledge. On the contrary, sometimes what is involved is the house officers' view that what they are expected to master by way of a data base and a repertoire of skills feels overwhelming. They are humbled by the parade of textbooks, scientific and clinical journals, grand rounds, case conferences, VIP lectures, and research colloquia that confront them daily, and are a reminder that medical school represented only the beginning of their medical education.

In the past, as students, the house officers have usually been told what to learn and when to learn it, even how to learn it. Those days are gone. Now as house officers they must be responsible for his or her own learning process and for internalizing a schema for acquiring basic information necessary to pass muster among peers as a competent specialist.

Classes may be few and far between; journal reprints are tossed to them with a brief word that what they contain must be learned; comments are made during ward rounds about new findings and new techniques being used, about which they may know nothing.

The house officers arrive home after a long day confronted with the need to study, yet probably too tired to learn anything new. They often feel guilty, inadequate, and sometimes incompetent.

Dr. McD., a senior resident in pediatrics, expressed it very well this way: "Maybe the underlying stress that's with you all the time is the nagging sense that you don't know enough. You keep fearing that you're basically incompetent, that things are going to come up suddenly that you can't handle. You never feel on top of everything in this business. You never have enough experience, and it's hard to maintain a consistent sense of self-confidence, although you go through periods when you're pretty high. Then, something happens, and you realize how much you don't know."

As Dr. Q., our otolaryngology resident, said, "I guess the major stress was one I didn't expect. The latest basic text on ENT contains 1,500 pages, and that is just the general text without all the subspecialty stuff, plus all the journals that come out every month. It's pretty overwhelming."

House officers may begin to wonder, as they compare themselves with their senior attending physicians whether their choice of medicine in general and of their specialty in particular have been good ones. They are constantly confronted by mounds of data that they are supposed to digest and use and, simultaneously, by the reminders (particularly through those of their patients who don't get well or don't get well quickly enough) of the shortcomings of their profession despite their struggles to master the information. This contrapuntal playing of the themes of their own inability to learn and master everything they need to know against the coda of the natural human limitations of the field of medicine often produces even more anxiety. House officers may have been convinced for years that if they could learn enough, fast enough, and well enough, they would enjoy the pleasures and triumphs of the accomplished physician. Perhaps now, for the first time in their lives, they are confronted with tasks they cannot fully master and are now humbled by the experience. There is nothing wrong with this, but they do not know it yet.

In the face of these confounding struggles, daily encounters with patients who do not behave as they "should" may leave house officers increasingly stressed. Patients and families who approach them with postures of exaggerated entitlement may leave them, in turn, angry, guilty, and then frustrated. They may feel that they are giving 150% of themselves to patients who are too demanding and, even so, are unappreciative.

For instance, there were the rather anguished complaints of Dr. R., the resident in obstetrics and gynecology, who stated very emphatically, "It isn't the patient with persistent complaints without organic pathology who gives me the most trouble. It's the extremely demanding patient who acts like the world owes her a living, the ones who expect special attention."

It was another OB/GYN resident, Dr. T., who made it clear how unsympathetic he felt toward women who complain "that this little pimple on her breast is a national emergency." He went on in great detail to talk about the mother whose baby had required electronic fetal monitoring and was now perfectly fine by all standards, although the mother was consumed with irrational fears that because "The baby looks funny to her and there is some trouble with his eyes, she thinks maybe he'll be blind as a result of this." The frustration with this kind of patient made Dr. T. reconsider for a time whether he wanted to continue this type of work. Then he felt reassured once more by all the very sick cancer patients he had to take care of.

Because of this, the house officer may spend excessive time with patients who have "irrational" complaints of mysterious symptoms, only to find that there is no biological explanation for them. When the patient's symptoms do not go away despite reassurances and explanations, the house officer may be even more enraged and end up feeling alienated from patients.

This risk of alienation may actually be increased in encounters with the most sick patients or the dying patient. The price for experiencing too much closeness carries with it such a potential burden of loss that an inevitable guarding and buffering of most emotions that serve to foster relationships will ensue.

Depending on what kinds of supportive attachments may have developed with the senior teachers, the house officer is also at risk of viewing them from afar and idealizing them, perhaps coming to see them as "iron men and women" who are fearless, tireless, and omnipotent. They may spend too many waking hours attempting to emulated teachers who, in their own understanding, have handled the terrible stresses that belabor physicians by learning how to become anxiety-free superpeople who are above it all.

The net result of this kind of process is that house officers are likely to get the least support from the people from whom they need it most; that they may hide their sense of deficiency and inadequacy so that these people will not be critical of them; and in the end, the house officers may therefore choose to go it alone without proper teaching supports. Thankfully, there were very few house officers in my sample who carried this to an extreme. Most enjoyed the risk of riding on the edges of their knowledge and skill, pushing themselves to the limit, making tricky clinical decisions, and asking for help only when they felt that they were moving beyond their resources in any serious way.

Virtually every house officer I spoke with talked about reexamining the choice to go into a particular specialty during the first year of postgraduate training. Almost all emerged from that period of reexamination feeling that, on balance, they had made the right choice and wanting to stay with it. This self-appraisal was triggered by the onslaught of "real" experiences in practice, which provided new insight against which earlier fantasies about the specialty could now be measured. Again, this is a healthy process but can shiver the timbers of any young person.

Dr. U., one of the neurology house officers, said as he began his second year of training, "This is the right field for me. The longer I'm in it, the more I like it. I knew I didn't like surgery. I like many things about medicine, but I liked everything about neurology. I knew I would fit in. I like the deductive reasoning, the precision of the neurologic exam, and getting the exact details of the history. And I'm basically happy with this residency because there's a lot of one-to-one teaching; it's small and compact. I came to the Northeast because I wanted to get away from the Southwest. Don't let these shitkickers fool you. [He held up one booted leg and laughed.] I'm not going back there."

Family practice residents, in particular, seemed to go through an intense period of self-examination during their first year of training. The idealism with which they had entered the program and the intensity of their commitment to work with families was sorely tested. Dr. N. came out of that year saying, "The fun of medicine is the people, the patients.

That's why I like the work in the family health center. I've gotten involved not only in their medical problems but in their total life situations." But Dr. F., at the same stage of training, said, "These experiences are causing me to rethink what I want to do when I'm finished. I told you my original choice was based on wanting to have long-term contact with families and to give comprehensive care. My mind is shifting on some of this. I'm finding out some things about myself in the process. I'm not enjoying the experience as much as I thought I would. It's not the patients so much; it's me. These long-term relationships with patients are not terribly rewarding."

Some house officers were actually reassured in a very positive sense through this critical period of reappraisal. Some even came to the realization that their choice of specialty had been based not only on factors of intellectual interest and personal skills, but just as importantly, on a preconscious awareness of their own temperamental attributes that would render them more likely to succeed in a given specialty and to fail, or at least to become unhappy, in another.

For instance, you may recall the comments of Dr. J., whose interview opened Chapter 4, and who said after his first year of training, "I just know that all the other specialties seemed dull and boring. There is something too routine about them. Psychiatry is much more exciting. I know the old story about every patient is different, but I watched internists and pediatricians and surgeons during my third-year clinical clerkships. They were all too rushed and too busy with gall bladders and kidneys and hearts to ever find out anything about their patients that made one different from the others. As I watched some of the faculty members in this department, that's a lot closer to what I want to be 10 years from now."

Dr. O., an ophthalmology resident in his second year of training, discovered this about himself: "I like the idea that ophthalmology is basically an outpatient office-practice specialty so you don't have to become involved in hospital bureaucracies. In some ways, I am sort of a loner, very independent. I don't like people telling me what to do, and you get into that if you have to work in a big hospital. I will do much better working by myself in private practice, although I wouldn't object to being part of a group. More and more hospitals dictate what you can or can't do with your patients, and I'm too much of an individual to live with that kind of system. Ophthalmology is a pretty discrete and separate specialty that doesn't really overlap with others like some do, so you have your turf marked out for you, and it isn't likely that other people are going to interfere with it. People value their eyes very much, and anything that is wrong with the eye tends to get people's attention, and you feel you are doing something for them that is valuable. Truthfully, I like working regular hours. I would never have a career where I couldn't have lots of personal time to do other things I wanted to do. In ophthalmology you can live that way. You are not a slave to medicine."

In some instances, there had been such a reverential attachment to a medical figure in the individual's life that the internalized image of the person carried the house officer through many bad experiences and many disappointments and remained a kind of beacon on the career pathway. Dr. I., our pediatric intern who gave birth to a baby during her first year of training, although highly critical of some of her attending physicians, said, "Having the baby brought me back to earth. Now I know we weren't ready to have a baby yet. I had worked and studied very hard for over 20 years, and I was headed for specializing in pediatrics. It was what I had always wanted. I had gone to med school for the express purpose of becoming a pediatrician. I guess a large part of it was the pediatrician who took care of us as we were growing up. I worshiped him. I still do. He is very proud of what I'm doing, and I keep in constant touch with him."

THE DILEMMA OF PERSONAL RELATIONSHIPS: SUPPORT OR CONFLICT

In addition to daily interactions with patients, every house officer is surrounded by a complex network of other human relationships. This network varies to some degree depending on the nature of the specialty, on whether he or she has a spouse and children, and on the size and organization of the peer group of trainees.

Regardless of these individual variations, however, it is safe to say that, in addition to patient contacts, there are three circles of interpersonal transactions taking place: one involving family; one involving clinical supervisors and attending faculty; and the peer group, made up of house officers in his or her own specialty and in others.

Although, in daily life, these would be difficult to consider completely independently of each other, it may be useful to do so here.

Kinship, Spousal, and Parenting Interactions

The table describing the demographic characteristics of our house officer group (Table 1, Chapter 1) lists two figures that, in themselves, may be rather surprising. These reveal the rather large percentage (57.7%) who are married and who have children (40.4%).

At the same time, there is little in these interviews about the house officers' families of origin, even though questions about this topic were asked routinely. Statistics concerning the percentage of house officers geographically separated from their families subsequent to a decision to train in a distant city are not included in the table because there were too many gray areas to permit such neat delineations. Often, there would turn out to be a brother-in-law, or an aunt, or a first cousin located in the city where training was taking place, and this permitted some contact with relatives by blood or marriage.

On the whole, however, most were not training in cities where they had grown up or where their parents and siblings were located. Yet, this received little of their attention in the interviews. The usual response was something equivalent to "Yes, I miss my family, but I wouldn't have much time to see them anyway even if I were located in the same city. We talk on the phone. They are proud of me and like what I am doing"—and so on. There was very little content that suggested that separation from family either added to the stress or created a major deficit in supports. This may have been related, as many house officers suggested, to the all-consuming nature of postgraduate training, but I suspect that an additional factor had to do with the developmental level of these young adults. Their career directions having been decided and their financial futures assumed to be reasonably secure, there was little need felt for parental closeness, counseling, or support. This would come later. New parent surrogates (their attending physicians) were now in place.

Relationships with marital partners and children presented a different situation, however. The house officers described many variations. Marriages in which one partner remained as the full-time homemaker presented one set of problems. Another was presented by two-career marriages and was seen in the most extreme circumstances where both were house officers. In a few instances, both partners were in training in different cities and saw each other on occasional weekends!

Dr. L., one of our residents in clinical pathology, was married to someone who was in training in another specialty. They had a two year old son. She described a part of their daily routine as follows:

▼   ▼   ▼

I realize now how much easier things would be without Timmy. Some nights, I have to pick him up at six o'clock if my husband can't get him, and that's a rush. He's in the university day-care center, and they charge you 5 dollars for every 30 minutes past six. It's nothing for me to be an hour or two late a few times a week. We can drop 50 dollars just like that. This medical center needs a day-care center just for the kids of house officers, so they can be dropped off and picked up at any time. If my husband has to go in at night and then I get an emergency call that I can't handle by phone, I go a little crazy trying to find someone to take care of Timmy in the middle of the night. When we're both on call, I try to have somebody sleep in, but that isn't always possible. Our evenings are pretty structured. We have to get dinner and there's a little time to play with Timmy, but then we have to get him to bed. Household chores get done around 9 or 10 at night. We try to get to bed before midnight.

Right now, there's no time or energy for any social life. It's pretty much just the three of us, at least for now. [Long pause.] When a woman has a career like this, there is no good time to have children. It wouldn't have been any better if we had waited. Then there are just other pressures and demands. I wish I had more time to spend with Timmy, but I also know that if I were with him all the time, I wouldn't be a better mother. Probably worse. I tend to get too uptight about things. He's better off spending good parts of the day away from me. Anyway, he seems to be doing fine.

▲   ▲   ▲

The news is not all bad, however. Some house officers reported marital relationships as positive, supportive, and playing an important role in buffering stress. Dr. L., a third-year resident in general surgery, said of his marriage:

▼   ▼   ▼

I have no regrets about getting married and having a family. You know that, in the end, it's only your family that will stick by you. Others will be for you or against you, depending on the winds of fate. The best stress coper in the world is having somebody who is willing to sacrifice for you. My wife and I are very conservative and have strong family values. We both come from that kind of background, and I know that, in the end, that's what's going to get us through. That doesn't mean she's not having a real rough time now. Everything at home is dumped on her: not just taking care of the kid and the housework but the repairs, the bills, the marketing—everything. I'm almost never available, and when I am there, I mostly sleep. She complains once in a while, but not much. Basically, she knew what she was getting into because I told her everything. I guess she had informed consent, but we both know that's worthless. There's knowing and there's understanding, and those are two different things.

▲   ▲   ▲

Perhaps the single most critical variable is not specific to the training itself but concerns the degree to which both partners anticipated what the experience would be like, discussed it openly and frankly, and came to some general agreement about what their mutual obligations would be during the training experience. In some ways, marriages in which there were two house officers in training were less stressful because each partner had an acute awareness of what the other was experiencing and what could reasonably be expected.

The observations of Dr. F., an unmarried second-year resident in neurosurgery, bear repeating. He saw the situation among his colleagues this way: "Some of the guys are having a lot of second thoughts. They're faced either with quitting the field or heading for separation and divorce. There's tremendous stress in their marriages because of their work load and their fatigue. Most of us can handle the stress of the training. There are very few surprises. We knew what we were getting into. Where it becomes unbearable is when you're involved with a wife or a fiancée. Those women are under a lot of stress themselves and, in the process, create a lot of stress for the residents. The minimum amount you have to do in neurosurgery training would be insurmountable for most people, but we do it. However, you can't give your loved ones what they need and deserve. They have to get along a lot more on their own. Among the residents, even among those who are not thinking of quitting the field, many are thinking of divorce because of the tension."

Marriages in which one partner came from a nonprofessional background or even a nonmedical background tended to be more tenuous because of the lack of sophistication of one partner concerning the demands of the residency. In any event, two-career marriages in which there were no children and in which the nonmedical partner was also extremely busy and often fatigued were sometimes less problem-filled because both spouses wanted to use time to rest and recuperate rather than to have long, intimate discussions, to enjoy recreational facilities, or to take active vacations.

In general, married female house officers had more difficulties because they were less relieved of household responsibilities than their male partners. Pregnancy and childbirth occurring during training presented very special problems for both partners. These difficulties were magnified if the department sponsoring the training proved to be unsympathetic to the needs of a pregnant family. Even the peer group of trainees who might be initially supportive and helpful to the pregnant trainee eventually became irritable and resentful as the ongoing pressure to pick up the absent member's work load became increasingly burdensome.

Perhaps one of the more extreme examples of this problem encountered during the interviews involved a young female house officer who became pregnant during her clinical pathology training. A colleague described the ensuing events as follows:

▼ ▼ ▼

Because of the exposure to AIDS, herpes, hepatitis, and the like, she wanted to be excused from autopsies until after she delivered. The other residents all discussed it, and we agreed to pick up her work load if she would take some extra on-calls later. At first, they said okay, but a few weeks later, they called her in and said no soap. She protested all the way up the university hierarchy, but the answer was still negative. In essence, what they told her was that she had signed up for this, and she would have to go through with it like everyone else. They told her if she didn't do the autopsies, then she'd have to leave the program. So she quit.

We were all very upset over this. She got no compensation. There just didn't seem to be any sympathy for her attitude. There have been several incidents like this.

▲ ▲ ▲

Perhaps the most accurate generalization that can be made about all of this is that postgraduate training tends to be a jealous partner, one that demands almost all of the individual's resources and that therefore also proves to be an isolating experience. The house officer may find herself or himself telling a spouse essentially that the patients come first; what little free time there is is necessarily consumed by the spouse, so that the trainee feels separated from her or his peers and, often, unable to partake of the social experiences that accompany training.

In discussing some of the positive and negative aspects of social life during training, Dr. S., a neurosurgery house officer, said, "You understand, I'm talking almost entirely about single people. Residents who are married and have kids have no social life whatsoever. The little energy you have remaining after a normal day goes into your family. For a while, my wife tried to get me to go out to some things, but I usually ended up falling asleep. She objected to that, so we stopped. We've stopped trying."

Even the "flex time" that might be available to the unattached house officer for reading and study generally could not be used by the married resident without running the risk of increasing marital tension.

Those house officers who were attempting to parent young children during training, of course, experienced additional pressures. Some, unfamiliar with the needs of infants and toddlers, were able to rationalize their own unavailability by stating that children at those ages really were not aware of the absence of a parent as long as one was available. They did not seem to experience much conflict about spending most of the time as absent parents. In the few instances where older children were present in the house, this was more difficult to explain away. Most often, the house officer proved to be reactive rather than proactive to the needs of older children, indicating that when the children were hurting or feeling needy, he or she would make every effort to respond to this.

Dr. Y., a 36-year-old psychiatric resident who described himself as a "retread" and who was the father of several older childen, said of them, "I worry about my own kids and what they're getting from me these days. Most nights, when I get home the two little ones are in bed already, although they are waiting up for me and we have a chance to talk for a while. The thing about my kids, though, is they have learned to be squeaking wheels and get the grease. If I neglect them too much, they let me know it in no uncertain terms."

Faculty and Attending Physicians

The most crucial relationships for these physicians in training, by common agreement, were with their teachers and supervisors. The inevitable love–hate relationships with the older faculty members who, in many ways, controlled their fate and also nurtured, mentored, and guided them toward future professional competence proved to be an oft-told tale. When you are approaching 30, it is difficult not to feel ambivalence toward an individual who may be in total control not only of your daily activities but of the future opportunities that may be open to you, and who, at the same time, shares with you his or her wisdom and experience and often provides support and counseling for you at difficult moments. It is a recrudescence of the most troubling developmental task of adolescence and hence strewn with pitfalls and land mines.

Dr. McD., a senior resident in pediatrics, in describing the kind of tensions that can develop between trainees and their clinical supervisors, had this to say:

▼   ▼   ▼

The attendings can have an enormous impact on your self-image. We all have attendings we don't like, but the real problem comes around attendings who treat you like you don't know anything. They kind of put you down and don't listen to what you have to contribute. They seem to show a lack of respect or interest in what your sense of the problem may be. That really upsets people. It's a lack of appreciation. It hurts to be ignored when you work so hard. Some attendings just have a bad attitude toward house officers. They don't trust them.

Private attendings are the worst because they have a tendency to have a low investment in teaching and in academics, and they want to get back to their offices. With some private attendings, there's almost a kind of hostility toward house officers. Maybe they feel we don't know what we're doing and these are their patients. It's circular. They have no interest in us, so we have a natural tendency to try to sock it back to them. We don't have the power to do that directly, so sometimes we take it out on the patient and the family which is very unfair and unreasonable. But the politics are such that you can't get rid of these attendings because the hospital needs them too badly to keep the beds full.

▲   ▲   ▲

Adolescents tend to grow incrementally as they come up against the reality that their parents are not simply authority figures but real people who have needs, too. The house officers in this sample struggled with this concept. Clearly, they most highly valued those attendings who were good clinical teachers, who were invested in the careers of their trainees, and who were willing to run risks by delegating the responsibility for clinical decisions and taking the rap when things did not go well. They were much less comfortable with the idea that the faculty members had careers of their own and that the reward system in teaching hospitals did not place teaching as the highest priority.

They were troubled about the fact that faculty members had to attract clinical and research monies in order to support their departments, and that they had to spend large amounts of time preparing research grants and carrying out research projects (which might seem of low priority to a house officer). Some felt cheated, even betrayed, by this priority system.

Almost to a person, they felt that the priorities needed to be shifted in most departments, with more emphasis on the importance of training and education. Many lived in fear of losing the best teachers. The following two quotations are representative of the dozens of comments that I heard. Dr. S., a second-year resident in neurosurgery, said,

▼   ▼   ▼

What I look for now is someone who is a sharp clinician and good technically in the OR, and someone who includes you in the decision-making process—someone who will give you support when you need it, especially if you're up against some attending in another department. There are a couple who fit that description, but there are several who don't. The former are my role models. We also have two other kinds of people in the department I don't go for. Some are just slow thinkers, or they don't think at all—they just make snap decisions and aren't very academic. And then, there are some who write good research grants and bring in a lot of research money. But they spend so much time doing research, I think they have lost some of their clinical smarts. Nevertheless, they are the ones who get the rewards.

The ones who are the best role models for the residents get lip service but don't get promoted and don't get any of the real goodies in the department. It's clear what the first priority is these days. When push comes to shove, it doesn't make any difference how good you are with the residents. Those attendings just get thrown the bones but they don't get any major rewards.

I think this attitude is pervading the whole medical center, and I think it's a big mistake. Ten years from now, the quality of the center won't be up; it'll be down as a result of this. All the good clinicians and teachers will have left.

▲   ▲   ▲

And there was Dr. M., the radiology house officer, who said, "I'm selfishly afraid that we are going to lose the four or five people we have who are genuinely interested in the residents. Maybe they will get too frustrated in trying to advance themselves and they'll move into private practice or other systems. Those people tend not to be squeaking wheels and don't get pushy about being advanced. They enjoy clinical work and teaching, and they don't look like superstars, but to the residents, they are worth their weight in gold."

Some house officers had little to say in response to some of the questions raised in this interview. Without exception, every house officer had comments to make about the criteria for a good attending physician (or a bad one) and what was expected from attendings in general. Perhaps the most universal response was that attendings were supposed to have a serious investment in the development of young people; to go out of their way to be helpful; and to demonstrate by word and deed that house officers were more than convenient labor and were major investments in the future of the specialty involved.

Although all of the interviews reproduced so far are laced through with comments about good and bad attendings, some house officers put it more succinctly than others. For instance, Dr. F., a senior resident in orthopedic surgery, was quite specific about his needs: "The things I look for first are what can I pick up in the OR by watching, you know, technique kinds of things. I look at surgical judgment, but I also look at how the attendings handle patients. Do they pay attention to them or are they just in and out and don't show much concern with how the patients are doing? Just the procedure itself? Most any attending can teach you something in a major disaster situation. The real test is, Can you learn some things in a more routine, straightforward situation that you didn't know before? That's a really good attending. Even though I'm a senior resident, I can still learn a lot from an attending. In this specialty, there are very few straight-arrow decisions. There are lots of judgment calls in terms of different options, and how you arrive at the decision is a thinking process you learn from good attendings. If you don't have that, it can be very tedious, and you feel like you are just putting in time and doing the things that other people don't want to do because you are a resident."

Dr. O., a senior neurology resident, summarized it briefly this way: "You look for an aura of confidence in an attending. It's what you identify with. It's what the patients look for. They want a doctor who conveys confidence and who doesn't come across as a wimp. The other thing you want in an attending is someone who is not so completely turned on by a research career that he or she doesn't spend a lot of time at the bedside with the residents."

As might be expected, residents wanted to admire their attendings, even to be in awe of them sometimes. They expected superlative clinical skills, and they wanted to be able to experience a sense of confidence in their attendings. Several indicated that they wanted their attendings to "inspire" them.

Many stated that it was important that attendings convey a reciprocal sense of trust in the house officers, in their competence, reliability, and intelligence. They felt they could not learn very much if they were overprotected and if attendings overfunctioned for them. At the same time, most wanted to be challenged, to be made to think, and to be stretched so that their performance would improve.

It is perhaps paradoxical that, despite the many stresses of training, most of these young people wanted to know their limits and enjoyed being stretched. Dr. J., one of the psychiatric residents from whom we heard earlier, said on this subject: "I've probably been exposed to maybe 15 or 20 attendings. I go for the ones that make me think out treatment decisions and keep me on target. I have a tendency to fly too much by the seat of my pants. The guy who brings me up short and forces me to explain my clinical decisions and helps me when my hand has been called and I can't is what I go for."

Dr. B., a senior radiology resident, unlike some of the house officers, complained about not being stretched enough: "I'm not being pushed hard enough or challenged. I look around me at house officers in most of the other specialties and they're busting their butts. You wanted to know how we cope with stresses, and I guess I'm saying that, like most people, I respond to pressure, and I'm not feeling enough of it to produce the way I should."

Almost all of the house officers appreciated rapid feedback, even if it was negative. It was helpful to know how one was doing and what needed to be fixed so that there was the best possibility of achieving what was expected. On the contrary, when feedback was long-delayed or even absent, this was viewed as a very negative process, one likely to result in uncertainty and even floundering.

One of the more common complaints by residents was that, although there might be a feedback system concerning their performance, it was subject to being filtered through the bureaucratic structure of the department, with results similar to those described by Dr. V., a house officer in emergency medicine: "There are evaluation forms filled out by each place we go to, but we don't get to see those until about three months later, and there is never any chance to discuss them with the attending who fills them out, so you don't really get a chance to fix your deficiencies while you are on a service. Anyway, a lot of the evaluation forms are very subjective. They really tell you whether you got along with somebody rather than what your strong or weak points were."

Sometimes, the evaluation system was seen as a *pro forma* procedure without real meaning. Dr. H., a senior resident in otolaryngology, described the system in his department as follows: "We do have regular evaluations at the end of each rotation. We are required to read them and sign off on them, and once a year we meet with the chief, who goes over these and chats with us about our progress. In general, though, if things are quiet, you assume you are doing well. No news is good news. More pats on the back, if properly earned, would help. Everybody is insecure in a residency, and you need signals about when you are doing well. I think they assume we know, and we don't always."

Some felt much resentment of what they considered tantamount to being treated as children by attendings. This was viewed as the epitome of distrust in the ability of house officers.

The attendings on whom house officers were likely to place the least value were those who seemed to be unable to delegate to subordinates or trainees and had to do everything themselves. Dr. D., a senior resident in internal medicine, voiced his pet peeve about attendings in this way: "One of the hardest things to do is to work with an attending who acts like he's in the 17th year of his residency. He's doing things exactly the way he did when he started. He has to take the blood pressure himself. He doesn't trust the intern. In fact, he repeats everything himself no matter what others have done. That's the worst kind of teacher, and we have some of those—unwilling to trust anything that anybody else does. And that kind of person is not going to change no matter what. The system of faculty supervision needs a fresh look. There's something wrong with it."

Besieged by their own sense of unreadiness and shaky self-confidence during training, these house officers felt especially vulnerable to demonstrations of lack of trust on the part of attendings. Dr. L., a surgical resident, said, "It's when you're not sure what to do that you might kick yourself afterwards. I guess it's just the business of growing up as a competent surgeon and feeling mature while, at the same time, you are trying to handle difficult attendings who treat you as a child when you are 30."

Dr. F., from whom we heard in the chapter on neurosurgery, highlighted the problem of distrust this way: "A lousy attending is one who takes over and you're nothing but a scrub nurse. There's nothing that a resident hates more than preparing for a case, going over all the studies, reading up the night before, and then not being allowed to do a darn thing on his or her own in the operating room."

Sometimes trainees found themselves functioning in ways that they judged to be role reversals. They might perceive the attending as being needy, immature, or such a prima donna that he or she had to be catered to or indulged. Worse yet, the attending might be seen as incompetent or failing to keep abreast of new developments, in which case the house officers might be expected to compensate for his or her deficiencies. Rarely was a full-time academic physician seen in this way, although it was not uncommon for so-called visiting or volunteer private-practice attendings to acquire this image among the house officers.

Dr. F., a fifth-year resident in orthopedic surgery, described his experience with role reversal this way: "Most attendings are pretty good, but in some places, you obviously have people who are not comfortable with some procedures in the OR and rely more on the resident than they ought to. It's a kind of role reversal where the resident has to keep an eye on the attending rather than the other way around. That's not what we're here for."

Dr. A., a third-year resident in otolaryngology, said of the situation: "There are a few attendings who we think are not terribly good among the private people. If they need a hand, we do assign somebody to them, but we make sure it's a senior resident who knows what he or she is doing and doesn't depend on the attending for the outcome. It ends up being a role reversal, with the residents sort of secretly supervising the attending."

Fortunately, these occurrences were not only rare, but apparently well known to the leadership of the department, so that safeguards were built in to protect both the patient and the resident in almost all instances.

In some specialties, interactions with senior attendings in other specialties (for instance, when anesthesiology house officers had to collaborate with senior surgeons) resulted in problems in maintaining the boundaries or the integrity of one's own specialty in the face of authoritative demands from a senior physician perceived as less expert in one's own area. This usually led to highly stressful situations. The house officers expected their own attendings to protect them from exploitation or misuse by going to bat for them. Attendings who were ineffective in this role were described as wimps.

Apparently, two types of house officers were most exposed to this problem. First, those in hospital-based specialties where the patient usually "belonged" to a physician in one of the medical or surgical specialties and the house officer and his attending were supplying collaborative services (e.g., anesthesia, radiology, laboratory services). There was a proclivity in such situations for one specialty to be dominated by another at the expense of professional self-esteem in the latter. The other situation in which this occurred was seen in such specialties as emergency medicine, where it was often necessary for the house officers to work in an environment where politics and procedures were controlled by other departments (e.g., internal medicine or surgery).

Attendings were observed more closely than they might have known in relation to how they communicated with patients and their families; how they made judgment calls about whether or not a patient should be admitted to the hospital; and, most of all, how they dealt with subordinates, secretaries, and nurses.

Two house officers whom we have already quoted expressed themselves succinctly on this point. Their words warrant brief repetition here. Dr. F., the orthopedic surgery resident, observed, "I look at surgical judgment, but I also look at how they handle patients. Do they pay attention to them, or are they just in and out, and do they show much concern with how the patients are doing?" And Dr. O., a family practice resident, put it this way:

▼   ▼   ▼

I watch how they make decisions about hospitalizing a patient, which patients really need hospitalization and which ones don't. Are they dumping the patient in the hospital because they don't have the persistence or the interest to really work the patient up carefully in the office and they want us to do the work for them? Or are they dumping the patient in the hospital for economic reasons because they will be reimbursed more if they round quickly on inpatients every day? You can tell, and these things make a difference.

You learn from both the positive and the negative. Either way, you begin to develop some very strong ideas about the kind of doctor you want to be—and the kind you don't want to be.

▲   ▲   ▲

But the cardinal sin for an attending was consistently placing his or her own career before the needs of house officers. There seemed to be almost no amount of hard work, long hours, menial assignments, and verbal abuse that these young physicians would not tolerate if they were convinced that their attendings would "put out for them." The attendings who were demanding, authoritarian, or even tyrannical at times could be endured if they provided opportunities for the resident to assume clinical responsibilities with difficult patients under close supervision—and if only once in a while they said, "Nice job."

Peer Group

As might be expected, the peer relationships in a postgraduate training program vary depending on the specialty and the size of the program. For instance, in some specialties, the trainee has comparatively little contact with others and works almost in isolation, depending more on interactions with attendings, technicians, nurses, and others. This might be true in clinical pathology, for instance, or in dermatology. On the other hand, in other specialties, particularly in surgical areas, there is a complex hierarchy of relationships reaching down from the chief resident to the most junior interns. In these situations, the relationships may even take on a more formal organizational quality, with the chief resident having some administrative responsibilities for the activities of her or his junior colleagues.

All of these situations have their pluses and minuses. In the tight hierarchical structure of a large surgical program, the more junior people champ at the bit, feeling that their progress is impeded by the needs of the more senior "siblings" who get the most difficult cases, perform the most complex procedures, and have the most time off. Some see this as akin to hazing the plebes. Yet, this structure provides considerable security, support, and guidance for beginners, a fact they often overlooked in their zeal to be handed the scalpel.

Dr. R., one of the OB/GYN residents from whom we have already heard, put the problem this way: "The senior resident decides what you get, and if you're low man, like I am, it's the leftovers. I guess if I have any complaint about this residency, it's the rigid hierarchical system between the years. The borders and territories are marked off by way of privileges and power, and you'd better not step over the boundaries. It chafes a bit. Sometimes, you offer to pitch in and help with something, and instead of being rewarded for being a good team player, you're scolded for stepping on somebody's toes."

As always, there is an informal and unwritten social structure in most training groups. This may function quite well in many situations, particularly if a resident has extra family responsibilities, needs extra time off because a parent has become gravely ill, or has other time-limited needs to which the group can respond collectively. Dr. V., one of the emergency medicine house officers, said of his peer group, "One of the major supports in this residency is that, within a given year, the resident group is very close. We do things together, trust each other, and have a lot of social life together. There is a lot of interchange at night and in the morning when you hand over the radio. We bitch to each other and complain and talk about the hard things that happened to us on the shift." And one of his colleagues added, "If it's a holiday or a special occasion and one of our guys is married and has a family, it's no problem to pinch-hit for him. We say 'Go on home. Be with your family. Everything will be okay.'"

"In more serious situations, which may involve drug or alcohol abuse, serious emotional disturbance, or emerging incompetence, the informal system may sometimes work counter to the needs of the trainee. Dr. Y., one of the psychiatric house officers, had very strong feelings about this situation and went into some detail, describing the anticipated fate of two of his colleagues as follows:

▼   ▼   ▼

As I look around me now at some of the other trainees in this program, I see some people having a very rough time. We talk about it among ourselves, but there is nothing we can do. They need help and are not asking for it. There's one guy who's almost paranoid about the administration of the hospital. He's so bound up with suspicion about how he's being exploited and so busy avoiding what he sees as extra responsibilities that he's not producing. Another one is quite depressed and is using alcohol too much—and he's become very expert at covering up both his depression and his drinking.

What are we residents doing about this situation? Some are looking the other way because they feel it's none of our business and they don't want to get involved. Others are covering up for these people by secretly picking up some of their work load. I don't know which is worse.

But I can guess from experience what's going to happen in the end. Things will progress to the point of no return before they're recognized by the administration. Both of these guys will have deteriorated far below the minimal level of acceptable performance in this place; they'll be put on probation; they won't be able to make it; and their contracts won't be renewed for next year. The first resident I mentioned will then go out and find himself a lawyer and sue the hospital, and the other one will get even more depressed and end up in the hospital, this time as a patient. How can this happen in a place like this, with some of the best trained psychiatrists in the world? I guess it's just the old story of the cobbler's children walking around with holes in their shoes.

▲   ▲   ▲

There is no escaping the fact that a medical department and its trainees share many features with the family. Without carrying the analogy too far, there are parental figues who are supposed to exercise some authority; to provide guidance and support; to behave in a differential manner toward the young, identifying and responding to the needs of each selectively; and when necessary, to mediate differences between the "siblings." In departments that operate smoothly and efficiently, these functions are carried out consistently. The fact remains that, in any family, whether related by blood or by professional interest, the resources are finite. This means that all involved must compete for both the material and the emotional goods that are available. For the house officer, this means competing for the time and attention of the attending; for access to the most interesting clinical cases; for opportunities for new learning experiences; and, finally, for opportunities to advance, such as promotion to chief resident or to a fellowship or perhaps even to a faculty appointment.

Because of these facts of life, there is an inescapable undertone of tension within a group of house officers that may stand in the way of their achieving trusting intimacy with each other.

Many training progams, aware of this undercurrent and of the considerable resource for buffering tension and stress that resides within the peer group, have developed approaches aimed at enhancing the strength of the group to serve its individual members. I will have more to say about this later.

Chapter 19

ENVIRONMENTAL STRESSES

What about the more mundane slings and arrows of everyday life in the teaching hospital? Our house officers have already described, or at least alluded to, a great many of them. To the interested onlooker, to the patient and his or her family, perhaps even to the hospital administrator who is not directly involved in patient management, these may appear to be the more important problems associated with postgraduate medical training.

Certainly, they are very real and quite serious and, in the extreme, may significantly interfere both with patient care and with the resident's learning experience.

Among the many we have heard about are chronic fatigue and sleep deprivation; concerns about financial indebtedness; time management problems, especially those connected with attempting to preserve some part of the day for personal life; "systems" problems related to hospital administration and the delivery of medical care; the intramural political conflicts of academic departments; and problems related to subsequent subspecialty choice and career planning, to name just a few of the most important ones.

A considerable amount of prior study of these areas has been carried out by medical administrators and faculty members in the past. There is much to be learned from these studies. They are summarized as a part of the literature review on this subject in Chapter 20 of this book.

Perhaps it is best to summarize and illustrate what my sample of house officers had to say on the subject. Although what follows in this chapter must inevitably be contaminated by my own past experience and by what I have read, I have done my best either to let these house officers speak for themselves or to attempt to collate and summarize what they said collectively about these matters.

CHRONIC FATIGUE AND SLEEP DEPRIVATION

As this is being written, the electronic and print media, together with professional journals and newsletters, are carrying major stories having to do with the so-called 36-hour day. The media presentations have a semisensational quality to them, suggesting that young house officers are forced to work like slaves for next to nothing doing the front-line work of unavailable attending physicians, very often to their own detriment and that of their patients.

Legislatures in several states have either passed or are considering bills that would regulate house officer hours in order to prevent supposed abuses. In general, there seems to be a disregard on the part of legislators and their staffs of the mechanisms now in place for the regulation of training programs, the licensure of hospitals, and the certification of medical care. Undoubtedly, there have been abuses. As interns and residents have complained since the beginning of such training programs, so have ours. No one relishes long, hard, and sometimes frustrating work days. This is particularly true if the work is viewed as not very remunerative. As the reader may have noted, most of our house officers were not impressed that this was the primary problem in their training.

In fact, Dr. O., whose interview begins the chapter on general surgery, was almost disdainful of house officers who "hung around" and were not efficient enough to get their work done quickly, particularly after a night on call. You may recall his words: "If you're observant, what you learn is that most people don't work the hours they tell you they do, nor do they need to. There's no need to be in the hospital until 9 or 10 every night if you are really organized, diligent, and efficient. There is too much hanging around the hospital. There's too much of this showing your face and being around in order to earn brownie points."

Dr. V., one of our neurosurgical house officers, had several interesting comments about the problem of fatigue and the on-call schedule. His points are instructive because they emphasize that, although the work is no Mediterranean cruise, adaptation takes place with a minimum of disruption of patient care. He put it this way:

▼   ▼   ▼

What happens after the first month is that you get into a pattern where you never feel quite right. Actually, that goes on whether you're on call every night or, as a junior resident, on call every third night. You kind of get used to always feeling vaguely nauseated and light-headed and not quite well. If you can get out of the hospital for a part of the night and spend time in your own environment and your own bed, your clinical judgment stays intact. There's something about being a prisoner in the hospital for days and nights at a time and being kind of totally separated from your other life that does impact on your judgment after a while.

There are plenty of people available when you're on alone at night if you want to call them. You simply have to recognize when you're in over your head and need help. That is a matter of watching yourself and knowing yourself. Some people do that better than others. I think I'm pretty good about that. You almost always have time to think things out anyway. There are very few occasions when you have to do something immediately at night. You have to order studies and usually get a CT scan so you have a minimum of 45 minutes to decide whether you want some help.

▲   ▲   ▲

Dr. T., one of the obstetrics and gynecology residents, said along these same lines, "The day after I'm on night call, I have to be especially on guard. I kind of feel like dog meat. I try not to make any quick decisions, and I try to consult more with other people. I don't want to make any mistakes."

Even in a worst-case scenario, there appeared to be, in most situations, a good many fail-safe mechanisms operating. Dr. F., an orthopedic surgery resident, said about his on-call experiences in one of the trauma hospitals, "If the next day you feel so spaced out that you can't keep your head about you and it is a very tough case and you may be with an attending who is not A+, you have to speak up. Maybe the chief resident can come in and help; maybe the attending can do it alone with an intern; maybe the case has to be canceled or postponed because you can't stay awake or you feel you don't have your wits about you. It's not fair to the patient if you don't say that. It usually works out, because if you are not functioning well, you can get some help, but if you keep it a secret, you can get into bad trouble. What I remember most about that experience is the kind of self-trauma that you impose. There is no time for any other life, personal or social or recreational. You either work or sleep. Little things like a good meal become of paramount importance to you, and you look forward to them.

There are certainly times when the vigor of the young physician is at least partially compromised; when perception becomes a bit fuzzy; and when the thinking process becomes slower. The reassuring aspect of this for me was the frequent statement that, for the most part:

1. The average house officer was particularly vigilant about the possibility of judgment errors when on night call or during the next day.
2. These house officers had encountered very few instances in which they had been called to task for misjudgments; rather, they understood that extra thinking time was necessary under such circumstances and that, because genuine emergencies requiring split-second decisions were rare, such time was usually available at no cost to the patient.

3. They had learned to judge the limits of their capacity and to ask for help either from peers or from attendings when they felt too stretched or too befuddled to think quickly and accurately.
4. In almost all specialties, this difficult time was restricted to one or, at the most, two years. It involved the internship and sometimes the first year of residency, as these are the times when the on-call schedule is primarily filled by junior house officers; once they had passed this period, their on-call responsibilities were attenuated or nonexistent—or could be covered from home by telephone on second backup call.
5. Most felt secure, because of their age, their vitality, and their resiliency, in handling the on-call schedule and in bouncing back rather quickly, with the understanding that attending physicians who were considerably older might have lost some of those qualities with the march of time.

Another aspect of all of this that seemed most striking was the self-selection process that took place. Individuals who needed eight or nine hours of sleep knew this by the time they were in their 20s and had not selected neurosurgery as a career. Specialties appeared to have been selected not only because they presented intellectual and/or financial rewards, but because of the lifestyle issues involved. Most of these features are known in advance by medical students and play a very important part in the decision about the specific nature of the professional practice in which they will be engaged for the rest of their lives.

In summary, although many house officers complained about being tired, especially during the early years of training, I can think of no instance in which this was viewed as more than a second-level and transient problem. The most typical attitude was one that viewed the long work hours as "coming with the territory" and as part of paying the dues for achieving the right to function autonomously as a medical specialist in the future.

FINANCIAL PROBLEMS

Most house officers reported that, by the time they were well into their training, their educational and personal indebtedness was substantial. Many were between $40,000 and $50,000 in debt. Some had spouses who were gainfully employed and assisted with the financial burden. If there were children, much of that extra money went for child care during the usual working hours.

None of these house officers seemed to be losing sleep over their financial status. The pressure they felt was to get on with their training, although some who entertained the possibility of a fellowship for subspecialization hesitated to do so because that would prolong or increase their indebtedness. All seemed to feel that, within three to five years, they would be able to satisfy their debts and to get on with improving their station in life.

Many reported that, although it would be nice to have more money, there was so little time for any personal life that it was unlikely that they could enjoy any of it. I do not mean to discount the importance of financial concerns during training. It is simply that none of these trainees seemed overly preoccupied with their present financial situation. Some who had small children regretted not being able to provide greater advantages for them currently, but all saw light at the end of the financial tunnel.

A particular problem that has arisen recently concerns the fact that federal regulations regarding the schedules for paying back federal educational loans now require that the process begin no more than three years beyond formal matriculation. Because many residencies extend four or more years beyond medical school, some residents are finding that they must begin to pay these loans back while they are still in training. This does create a significant fiscal squeeze on their domestic budgets and may create greater pressures to moonlight. If these pressures become excessive, further problems with sleep deprivation and fatigue may ensue.

TIME MANAGEMENT AND LIFESTYLE CONCERNS

In the never-ending cycle of on-call schedules, new patient assignments, seminars, lectures, rounds, and emergencies, many house officers had almost declared a moratorium on achieving any kind of gratification outside of the hospital beyond the simple, primitive pleasures of eating and sleeping.

Many who had been accustomed to active social lives in college and medical school felt rather deprived and isolated in the relentless hospital environment, restricted solely to the relationships they could develop with their training peers.

In terms of time and energy commitments, marriage and children proved, as one might expect, to be a two-edged sword. Dr. G., a psychiatric house officer and a father and husband, said,

▼   ▼   ▼

Between my work schedule and my family life, the academic stuff tends to suffer. Sometimes, I envy the unmarried residents because they can go home at the end of the day, and if they decide to read journals, they can do it. I can't, but there is no way I would trade what I've got. I won't pretend that marriage and parenthood haven't produced a lot of conflict for me. There are too many things I want to do, but the evenings are pretty much like the days. Two evenings a week, I see outpatients and get home very late. Two evenings, my wife goes to class, so she picks me up about six and we drop her off, and then I take care of the baby until she gets home. All day Saturday, I moonlight at a community mental-health clinic in the suburbs.

We joke about it. Some nights, we look like a pro football team doing double reverses passing the baby off to each other as we cross going to different places.

We don't have much social life, but we don't want much. We have so little time together that an unscheduled evening or two is something we want to spend alone together—just we and the baby.

▲   ▲   ▲

Many chafed under the rigors of their new life, which no longer permitted regular exercise, entertainment, recreational reading, or the pursuit of avocations. Yet, most had learned how to make adjustments and compromises so that at least some small piece of a prior life could be sustained. One intern exercised at the expense of taking her car in for needed repairs: "I get to work about 5:30 A.M. everyday, and during warm weather, I bicycle in. I guess I would have to do it anyway, since my car is on the blink and I've had no time to get it fixed. It just sits in the street. It's a big problem to take care of anything personal because there is very little flexibility or free time, and what little free time there is, I like to use for 'play,' like tennis or something."

Another listened to classical music some evenings instead of reading professional journals (obviously, listening to classical recordings did not constitute background music for him). Still another found time to be on the long-distance telephone to family and friends in his home city, although this telephoning cut deeply into what little free time he had for other activities.

Some indicated that it mattered little what they did as long as it was outside the hospital and free from binding schedules. Hospital life was seen as monastic and socially isolating—not so good for one's mental health. Dr. V., the neurosurgical resident whom we quoted earlier in this chapter, made it very clear that, for him at least, being out of the hospital in a different environment for a while made him think more clearly, even if it was only to spend a few hours in his own bed at home.

Once more, it was the time-limited aspect of this period that permitted many to survive and to fantasize about another day, when they would have more control over their own schedules and when other, younger house officers would do their "donkey work" so that they could go to the theater, spend time with their families, and play tennis.

SYSTEMS PROBLEMS

Even a casual reading of many of the interviews that have appeared so far will underscore the observation that the hospital administrators were not highly favored by these house officers. They were variously described as "the green eyeshade guys," "the bean counters," or the "executive suite mafia."

They were viewed with suspicion and distrust. Apparently, when they were doing a good job, little or no notice was paid to them. When they were seen as interfering with the house officer's freedom to do what seemed right at the moment, they were seen as bumbling bureaucrats. In all of the hours I spent with these house officers, I never heard a kind word for a hospital administrator.

Inevitably, these often distant authority figures served as convenient scapegoats for young physicians who were troubled (at what felt to them like advanced ages) with needing to be controlled by people who knew little or nothing about medicine.

Most saw nothing creative or original in performing administrative tasks, even in designing a medical care system and making it work. At best, it was seen as a necessary evil imposing restrictions on physicians even in areas they viewed as sacrosanct (who might come into the hospital; how long the patient might stay if he or she came in; what equipment would be purchased and where it would be placed in the hospital; when patients might be deemed eligible to be relieved of costs and when they might not be; and so on). They viewed all of these matters as requiring medical judgment, and they saw the authority of the administrator as usurping that of the physician.

Some of the more senior house officers believed that they should be consulted more, even in the areas of administrative and policy matters. They saw themselves as knowledgeable professionals and wanted to have significant input into decisions about the selection of chief residents, the appointment of department chairpersons and the content of the benefit packages for trainees. For instance, we previously heard Dr.

L., a surgical house officer, say, "Recently, they have been talking about cutting some of our benefits because of fiscal problems. No one asks us which would be the easiest ones to give up. These stresses are even worse because you are an adult, a husband, a father, and virtually a surgeon, but many people treat you like you're a kid."

Another systems issue that was quite stressful for some involved sharing the clinical decision-making process with team members in other disciplines. They tended to view life as simple for the autocratic surgeon in the operating room whose every command was obeyed without question. Most had not yet acquired the executive and diplomatic know-how to manage a complex team and would clearly have preferred to have a pyramidal authority system in which the decisions filtered down from the top. Yet, in another context, most would have agreed that, in this world of superspecialization, no physician has all of the knowledge and skills that a team can bring to diagnosis and treatment, especially if the team includes people like clinical nurse specialists, physical therapists, speech pathologists, clinical psychologists, and family counselors.

Dr. Y., a psychiatric resident who explained that part of the reason for his leaving the field of internal medicine was his sense of isolation in solo practice, said, "It's funny, but now when I get home at night, I'm just as tired as before, maybe more. Some of it is the flip side of the isolation I was feeling in practice. In this job, you end up praying for five minutes to be alone. The number of high-powered professionals I have to work with every day is probably close to 30 or 35. I'm not complaining, because it's what I really wanted, but sometimes, even the names get to be a problem. Each one has his or her own perspective on the patient. It's hard to figure out whom to listen to and whom you can't pay much attention to because they lead you down blind alleys and detours. As the M.D., you have to bring all this together and make it work for the patient. When I'm new on a service, I spend a fair amount of time comparing notes with other residents to see how they are sorting out information. If we agree on the same people who are giving us a lot of static, then I know it's not me, and I tend to downplay their input."

Much time is spent in chasing down laboratory values and other diagnostic studies on patients. Because of the short length of stay in hospitals at this time, there is no longer the luxury of waiting until the results of studies filter through a complicated communication system. Junior house officers become gofers, running to radiology, to clinical pathology, and to special laboratories to track down the results of consultations, biopsies, or blood studies done earlier in the day or at a previous time, in the hope of assembling all the necessary information before attending rounds. This takes enormous amounts of time on the telephone or "on the hoof," especially in a large multispecialty hospital.

Our house officers were particularly critical of hospital administrators who failed to recognize what they believed to be inefficiency or lack of interest on the part of the "gatekeepers," that is, the staff members who attended to the front door, reception, registration, financial interviewing, and all the other stations that had to do with entering a new patient into the system. You may recall Dr. U., a second-year resident in neurology, who said, "There is horrendous management, extremely inefficient personnel. It takes forever to get anything done or to get a patient through the system. At the VA, the physical facility is the pits, but the nurses are on top of things. They move the patients through at an incredible rate; yet, nobody feels rushed or neglected. And at another hospital we rotate through, it's also very efficient, but at our own university clinic, things just don't run well. You waste a lot of valuable time just sitting around waiting for patients to be 'processed.' I don't know what they're doing with the patients, but I don't see anybody hustling."

And there was the ophthalmology resident who said of another hospital where he worked, "The residency is fine. I don't see a need for any significant changes there, but I would fire all the people the first chance I got that had anything to do with greeting patients at the door — doing the paperwork, doing the financial interviewing, doing the reception. They are cold, bored, and uninterested and make everybody feel unwelcome. No matter how good the rest of the staff is, if that first person you meet when you walk in the door doesn't handle you right, you have a sour taste in your mouth. Nobody smiles. They look up at the patients as if they are interfering with their work."

Especially in pediatric settings, house officers in the surgical specialties felt on guard against many of the nurses, whom they saw as overprotecting the patients against the mean, invasive doctors. They believed that these systems problems were not adequately dealt with either by the hospital administration, the nursing department, or the pediatric physicians. Dr. F., a neurosurgery resident whose interview is reproduced completely at the beginning of Chapter 9, was eloquent in his indictment of pediatric personnel. He viewed their maudlin investment in their small patients as interfering with good care rather than facilitating it. His first choice would have been to start cleaning house by firing the entire nursing staff in the pediatric hospital.

Many systems issues that might seem to cause difficulty, in general, did not. Most trainees rotated between hospitals, each of which had different policies and practices requiring adaptation each time a resident rotated in or out. Complaints about this kind of thing were minor because most trainees felt more than compensated by exposure to different attendings, different patient populations, and a different focus on clinical practice.

POLITICAL AND TURF BATTLES

We have come to know that it is a myth that children do not know about the "secret" conflicts of their parents. This is even more true in the teaching hospital, where, inevitably, the large egos possessed by service chiefs, departmental chairpersons, hospital directors, and others walking the corridors of power may collide with one another on a daily basis.

Although the "offspring" may be aware of these battles, they rarely understand the basic issues involved because they are not privy to the intimate discussions, nor are they developmentally prepared to grasp the significance of what they may hear.

Yet, there is no denying that any major conflict between the decision makers in a group may have a significant impact on its most junior and dependent members. As Dr. H., the pathology resident, said in quoting one of his attending physicians, "When the elephants fight, the grass dies."

Sometimes, our house officers' welfare was not directly involved. They suffered only indirectly because the attending physicians took sides, a significant portion of their energy became consumed in the conflict, and the needs of the trainees dropped a few notches on the priority scale.

At other times, the residents saw themselves as being victimized more directly because of the turbulent political climate. They believed that this occurred when departmental heads engaged in mindless battles for power over a clinical area or a special activity. For instance, emergency medicine residents saw themselves as caught in the conflict between their own chiefs and those in medicine and surgery, who attempted to maintain administrative control over hospital emergency rooms.

Dr. V., one of the neurosurgical house officers, was particularly disturbed because a fellow trainee was virtually ignored when he had done an outstanding piece of research under the tutelage of the "wrong" professor, that is, one who was in disfavor with the chairman of the department. He added, "These sorts of issues leave me with very mixed feelings about my own career. There is some long-standing conflict with many of the leaders here and no one knows why. Maybe they don't even remember themselves anymore. Maybe it's just turf, but it creates a lot of unnecessary stress for the full-time faculty. It seems to make them dour. They lose their sense of humor and they get stuffy and self-important. I don't know that our department is different from others. They are probably all this way, more or less."

A related example may occur when shifting philosophical positions result in certain types of attending physicians' enjoying higher levels of reward than others. Many residents perceived that, in the climate of the 1980s, science rather than clinical teaching was the commodity that would bring the highest selling price. Therefore, attending physicians, in their eyes, were being courted if they were expert researchers and could bring in grant funds, at the expense of attending physicians who were good clinical mentors and supervisors. For a more detailed discussion of this problem, please see the section on attending physicians in Chapter 18.

Several house officers seemed so troubled and threatened by what they described as "academic politics" that, although they expressed some interest in research and teaching as a career, they planned to eschew a career in academic medicine because they did not want to contend with or could not compete with such an environment.

NEED FOR EARLY SPECIALIZATION

Many house officers felt considerable pressure, particularly if they were training in a specialty in which there was a physician oversupply, to make very early decisions about subspecializing in order to ensure financial security. Another reason to make such an early decision was to apply for and receive a fellowship in a desirable hospital setting.

In any event, the need to make decisions about what would prove to be a lifelong professional activity after a very short period of time in training placed many trainees under what they perceived to be premature and unnecessary pressure. They believed themselves to be making such decisions based on inadequate experience and for reasons that were far from educational in nature.

They saw the net effect as restricting their horizons, narrowing their approach prematurely, and forcing them into practice patterns that might prove in the future to be incompatible with their long-range interests or their own temperamental characteristics.

SUMMARY

House officers appear to suffer from the same work stresses that most people do: fatigue, financial problems, time management, organizational rivalries and conflicts, and concerns over long-range career plans. Viewed in isolation, these may be only quantitatively different from the everyday problems of the average working person. Placed in the context of the demands of training in an environment that frequently involves life-or-death decisions and interventions, they have to carry

more weight. For those of us who must be concerned about either planning programs for these physicians or consuming their services, these
stresses may take on special meaning. We run the risk of overemphasiz-
ing their importance because they will easily lend themselves to logical
solutions (e.g., limiting on-call hours), or we may underemphasize their
importance because we, too, have fallen prey to the myth that physicians
are superpeople and are therefore above the travails to which mere mor-
tals succumb.

Chapter 20

BACKGROUND AND LITERATURE REVIEW

INTRODUCTION

It was not until a few centuries ago that the teaching of the healing arts was formalized into a planned curriculum. Although there are some earlier examples, many European universities did not develop faculties of medicine as integrated components of their academic organizations until the 16th or 17th centuries. In the United States, this evolution did not occur, in most instances, until the 19th century, when Harvard University, the University of Pennsylvania, and Johns Hopkins University led the way in this regard.

I am, of course, referring to the undergraduate study of medicine. It was not until the 20th century, occasioned by the explosion of scientific information and a proliferation of specialties and subspecialties, that postgraduate training became formalized into what we now know as residencies and fellowships in the United States. Hence, there is not a long history over which the evolution of these postgraduate programs can be studied and their contributions and problems understood.

Until the 20th century, the basic teaching of medical practice on the North American continent was considered so primitive by European professors that many saw American physicians as charlatans or medicine men. In the first exhaustive historical review of medical education, Puschmann,[1] a Viennese professor, stated of American medical education, "Some medical schools enjoy, and justly so, a high reputation... along with these, however, there exist others which occupy a low position both intellectually and morally. The scandalous traffic carried on by many faculties in doctors' diplomas is well-known. ...It is, therefore, not a matter for surprise that American degrees in medicine should be regarded with distrust in Europe and placed in the same category as those amiable but meaningless distinctions which are conferred on people dancing the cotillion" (pp. 534–535).

On invitation from the Council on Medical Education of the American Medical Association, the Carnegie Corporation commissioned Mr.

Abraham Flexner in 1908 to conduct an objective survey of medical education in the United States. Mr. Flexner spent two years visiting virtually every medical school in the country. His famous report[2] on the findings of this survey proved to be the catalytic agent that stimulated a revolution in American medical education.

Substandard schools were closed, curricula were made more uniform, entrance requirements for students were elevated considerably, and universities, in general, began to exercise more careful scrutiny of the conduct of their medical faculties.

This process not only played a major part in advancing the teaching of medicine but also accelerated the pursuit of formal scientific research based in medical schools. Indirectly, it resulted in the growth of American medicine and in its later proliferation into many specialties.

By the second and third decades of the 20th century, most specialties had developed formal residencies or fellowships, although these were not, at the beginning, required for certification. The emergence of major teaching hospitals in Boston, New York, Philadelphia, Baltimore, and Washington, all affiliated with prestigious schools of medicine, created a clinical and educational environment in which postgraduate medical education could thrive.

The importance of the teaching hospital cannot be overemphasized as a force in improving educational standards, both in undergraduate and postgraduate medicine. Glaser[3] pointed out that, until the turn of the 20th century, undergraduate "students saw little or nothing of patients and were expected to gain clinical experience only after they received the M.D. degree" (p. 22).

Because specialty training, unsophisticated as it was, took place largely on an apprenticeship basis in the doctor's office, major teaching hospitals were not highly valued until the 20th century. Glaser stated that it was "the development of the forerunners of internship and residency which have become such a key part of medical education. . . . In New York at the Bellevue Hospital, among other institutions, there developed the forerunner of the modern house officership. Around 1900 the so called graduate programs began to be emphasized on a major scale" (p. 23). It was at Johns Hopkins that William Osler and William S. Halsted served as the first professors of, respectively, medicine and surgery, pursuing the model that they had seen in German clinics. They adopted this overall approach at Hopkins. This served as a kind of prototype for other major university programs (pp. 23–24).

From these comparatively recent and very modest beginnings, there has emerged, during the past 75 years, a very complex and sophisticated system for training young physicians in specialties and in subspecialties leading, usually, to certification by one of the specialty boards approved by the Accreditation Council for Graduate Medical Education.

At this writing, the latest Directory of Graduate Medical Education Programs (1987–1988)[4] lists 6,332 accredited graduate programs in medical education as of December 1986. The projection of positions for July 1987 was 79,854. This did not include physicians in 586 programs accredited too late to be included in the survey. In 1986, more than one fourth of the residents were women, and 38% of these were training either in internal medicine or pediatrics. The percentage of all residents who reported their race as black has remained at 4.5%. There were 1,343 hospitals offering a significant portion of training in graduate medical-education programs. In addition, there were 227 ambulatory care clinics, mental health agencies, blood banks, and medical examiners' offices that provided residency training (see Table 3).

HISTORICAL BACKGROUND AND RECENT PAST

There is surprisingly little in the literature pertaining to interns and residents before the early 1970s. There are many papers and volumes about medical student experience and education and about the medical profession and its activities. Between these, there is a kind of information hiatus about house officers, however.

In 1948, Brosin[5] and his colleague Earley attempted to follow 230 subjects who were studied as first-year medical students. Each was given a battery of tests and was directly examined by a psychiatrist. Efforts were made to predict their academic and professional success and their future personal adjustment. Although this was not *per se* a study of house officers, it was noteworthy in that it was one of the first formal attempts to measure outcome through personality and competence factors.

Aldrich[6] was able to locate 208 of these subjects almost 40 years later and reported on their status at the time in a recent paper. He concluded that "the psychiatrist's favorable predictions were, for the most part, borne out, whereas the unfavorable predictions were less likely to have been realized. The psychiatrists appeared to have overemphasized the significance of the psychopathology they discovered and to have underestimated the potential of many of these young adults for spontaneous personality change" (p. 45).

Becker and his colleagues[7] published the widely quoted *Boys in White: Student Culture in Medical School* in 1961. Again, this was primarily a look at the experience of undergraduate medical students (at the University of Kansas Medical School), and except for a chapter entitled "Student

TABLE 1

Number and Percentage of Programs and Residents on Duty
September 1, 1986, by Specialty[a]

Specialty	Number of programs	Percentage of programs	Number of residents	Percentage of residents
Allergy and immunology	87	1.4	244	0.3
Anesthesiology	164	2.6	3,864	5.0
Colon and rectal surgery	27	0.4	48	0.1
Dermatology	100	1.6	772	1.0
Dermatopathology	24	0.4	27	—[b]
Emergency medicine	69	1.1	1,203	1.6
Family practice	383	6.0	7,238	9.4
Internal medicine	442	7.0	18,116	23.6
Cardiovascular disease	212	3.3	699	0.9
Endocrinology and metabolism	141	2.2	158	0.2
Gastroenterology	178	2.8	332	0.4
Hematology (medicine)	154	2.4	172	0.2
Infectious diseases	149	2.4	216	0.3
Medical oncology	158	2.5	229	0.3
Nephrology	149	2.4	240	0.3
Pulmonary diseases	170	2.7	339	0.4
Rheumatology	116	1.8	132	0.2
Neurological surgery	93	1.5	719	0.9
Neurology	122	1.9	1,408	1.8
Nuclear medicine	91	1.4	176	0.2
Obstetrics/gynecology	290	4.6	4,525	5.9
Ophthalmology	142	2.2	1,549	2.0
Orthopedic surgery	168	2.7	2,822	3.7
Otolaryngology	107	1.7	1,090	1.4
Pathology	247	3.9	2,299	3.0
Blood banking	39	0.6	28	—[b]
Chemical pathology	2	—	1	—[b]
Forensic pathology	39	0.6	34	—[b]
Hematology (pathology)	12	0.2	5	—[b]
Medical microbiology	1	—	0	—[b]
Neuropathology	58	0.9	37	—[b]
Pediatrics	234	3.7	5,817	7.6
Pediatric cardiology	45	0.7	128	0.2
Pediatric endocrinology	49	0.8	66	0.1
Pediatric hemato-oncology	42	0.7	108	0.1
Pediatric nephrology	30	0.5	34	—[b]
Neonatal-perinatal medicine	99	1.6	350	0.5
Physical medicine and rehabilitation	70	1.1	817	1.1

TABLE 1 (*Continued*)

Specialty	Number of programs	Percentage of programs	Number of residents	Percentage of residents
Plastic surgery	95	1.5	401	0.5
Preventive medicine, general	28	0.4	199	0.3
Aerospace medicine	3	—	67	0.1
Occupational medicine	25	0.4	126	0.2
Public health	9	0.1	21	—[b]
Combined general preven- tive medicine/public health	8	0.1	68	0.1
Psychiatry	211	3.3	4,892	6.4
Child psychiatry	126	2.0	602	0.8
Radiology, diagnostic	215	3.4	3,095	4.0
Radiology, diagnostic (nuclear)	46	0.7	88	0.1
Radiology, therapeutic	86	1.4	499	0.6
Surgery	301	4.8	7,880	10.3
Pediatric surgery	19	0.3	32	—[b]
Vascular surgery	48	0.8	70	0.1
Thoracic surgery	95	1.5	286	0.4
Urology	132	2.1	1,043	1.4
Transitional year	182	2.9	1,404	1.8
Total	6,332	100.0	76,815	100.0

[a]Source: AMA Accreditation Council for Graduate Medical Education: 1987—1988 Directory of Graduate Medical Education Programs. Chicago, American Medical Association, 1987, pp 100. Reprinted with permission.
[b]Less than 1/10th of 1%.

house officers.

A more pertinent title appeared in 1970. This was by Emily Mumford,[8] a social scientist, and was entitled *Interns: From Students to Physicians*. Although the work is interesting and was timely, it can no longer be represented as reflecting the current experience of house officers as they make the demanding transition from student to house officer.

Indeed, Mumford made a special point of our tendency to ignore the experience and the special needs of house officers until recently. For instance, she pointed out that, in a 1962 bibliography in medical sociology, there are 18 titles on medical education but none specifically related to interns, residents, or their training programs. She indicated that the 1964 Cumulative Book Index reported several works on medical students, but nothing on interns or residents. As late as 1965, she indicated that the New York Public Library Catalogue had no entries for interns or residents, and that the Library of Congress had only eight entries, none of the work by social scientists (p. 234).

Knowles's[9] work on the teaching hospital (in which Glaser's already quoted chapter appears) was a significant milestone in putting before public view the important role and the dilemmas faced by teaching hospitals in the United States as the profession of medicine moved from the secure and certain role of the 1950s to the tumult and litigious environment of the 1970s and 1980s. Again, it does not focus specifically on the concerns of house officers as such.

CURRENT LITERATURE

Beginning in the early 1970s, there began to appear in the literature several papers directed more specifically at the experiences of house officers. Although some of these were "generic" in nature and strove for an overview of the issues, many began to direct our attention to concerns that either were specialty-based or were specific problems germane to the house officer experience (e.g., fatigue and sleep deprivation, financial matters, educational dilemmas, career planning, and adult developmental issues).

What follows is a brief overview of this literature. Citations that are specific to a particular specialty have, for the most part, been listed in the bibliography for that specialty earlier in this volume.

"GENERIC STUDIES"

In the 15 years between the early 1970s and the mid-1980s, there have been dozens of papers that address the general problems of (1) the transition from studenthood to physicianhood; (2) stresses and stress coping in house officers; and (3) the transition from residency to practice.

Early in the period, a volume by Coombs and Vincent[10] appeared, entitled *Psychosocial Aspects of Medical Training*. Even 17 years later, this work merits the attention of serious students of the field of medical education. It contains many chapters by outstanding authors in areas such as the transition to physicianhood, the virtues and the vices of specialization, and the careful observations of social scientists on postgraduate medical training as major teaching hospitals were about to launch themselves into a period of high-technology medical care unprecedented in the history of the professions.

About the same time, Vaillant and his colleagues,[11] who had been studying coping mechanisms, vulnerability, and their relation to health status in long-range projects involving populations of young men, published an interesting study entitled "Some Psychological Vulnerabilities of Physicians." Retrospectively, they looked at the childhoods of 47 physicians and compared them with those of 79 socioeconomically matched controls in occupations other than medicine. Physicians, especially those involved in direct patient care, demonstrated as a group less adaptive track records. They were more likely to have relatively poor marriages, to abuse drugs and alcohol, and to require at least outpatient psychiatric care. Vaillant and his coworkers pointed out that, although these difficulties are assumed to be occupational hazards of the profession, their presence or absence was rather strongly related to life adjustment before medical school. In other words, the most vulnerable physicians seemed to be those with the least stable childhoods and adolescent adjustments.

During the past decade, many other writers[12-24] have studied and described the variety of stresses encountered by interns and residents more-or-less independently of their particular specialty. There is general agreement in these papers about the nature of these stresses, although they may vary in degree, depending on the particular specialty and the year of training. In general, these include (not necessarily in the order of importance):

A. Interpersonal and developmental issues
   1. Marital, pregnancy, and parental concerns
   2. Attending-physician and faculty issues
   3. Patient-generated issues
   4. Career options and choices
   5. Depression, substance abuse, and suicide
B. Environmental stresses
   1. Financial problems
   2. Chronic fatigue and sleep deprivation
   3. Early specialization
   4. Systems issues

In addition, most of these writers pointed out the problems in dealing with rapidly altering mood states; especially bouts of depression and the temptations of dealing with stress through resorting to substance abuse continued to be major concerns for many house officers.

SPECIAL PROBLEM AREAS

The above papers tend to be broadly descriptive, and although they are generally helpful in understanding the scope of the problem, it is the more recent and more structured studies of specific problems encountered by house officers that are more informative and that tend to suggest a variety of approaches, both on the part of the house officers themselves and on the part of faculty, attending physicians, and hospital administrations. A brief review of some of this recent literature follows.

INTERPERSONAL AND DEVELOPMENTAL ISSUES

Marital, Pregnancy, and Parenting Concerns

Generations of impecunious house officers found it possible to pursue their training only in the single state. In my class of interns at the Philadelphia General Hospital in the 1940s, as I recall, only 4 of about 100 interns were married, and they had independent incomes. Also, in those days, most marriages were not two-career arrangements, so that the female spouse was rarely an independent generator of income herself.

Today, it appears that more than half of the house officers are married, and more than one third have children. Undoubtedly, this has relieved many tensions and created new support systems, but the price, especially for female house officers, can be very high.

Dena Lovett,[25] in a 1986 issue of *JAMA*, described in poignant and dramatic terms, using only six brief paragraphs, the plight of the intern's spouse. In capsule form, the burdens of geographic relocation, of long hours and days separated from one's spouse, of loss of friends and social interactions, of having to be virtually a "single parent," and of the multiple financial strains are starkly highlighted. Her questions resonate sympathetically with anyone who has been through the experience: "We dreamed of being so happy in our new home. Instead, we have found fear and loneliness. We have found the nightmare of internship. Does anyone care? Will anyone help?" (p. 3395).

Again, formal studies of this phenomenon are difficult to come by.

Because of their self-image, their striving for independence, and their concerns about confidentiality, it is very difficult for young physicians to seek help. Krell and Miles[26] suggested approaches in this regard. Gabbard and his colleagues[27] emphasized that, in their study, contrary to conventional wisdom, the number of hours at work did not relate to the degree of marital satisfaction. They reported that "lack of time due to the demands of practice seems to be a complaint that serves the function of externalizing the conflicts in the marriage cnto factors outside the marriage" (p. 571).

More recent studies emphasize the particular problems of female house officers who attempt marriage, and often motherhood, during their training. The vicissitudes of this particular lifestyle have been well explored by Kelner and Rosenthal,[28] Franco et al.,[29] Stewart and Robinson,[30] Sayres et al.,[31] and Coombs and Fawz.[32]

A firsthand account of this difficult and frustrating experience was described by Levy[33] in a brief piece in *JAMA* concerning her efforts to be surgeon, wife, and mother. She stated, "Let me tell you, once and for all, that this is neither physically nor psychologically possible. The myth is that a women engaged in a rewarding career—in any profession—can raise her children. Take my word for it, someone else is, call it Grandma, au pair girl, or day-care, call it anything but Mom" (p. 536).

Both the American Medical Association and its Ad Hoc Committee on Women Physicians in Organized Medicine[34] and the American Association of Directors of Psychiatric Residency Training[35] have approached this problem in an effort to stimulate training programs and hospitals to design policies that will be supportive of the pregnancy experience and of subsequent child rearing for couples in which one partner is in postgraduate training. There is no universally acceptable philosophy concerning this, nor is there a generally applied set of practices currently in force. Most training programs will provide some maternity leave (perhaps six weeks to two months). This is barely enough to permit the woman and her mate to get through the final days of the third trimester, the delivery, and the immediate neonatal period. Even so, the resident must confront often hostile attitudes among her peers because they are faced with picking up the slack of her work load in already tight schedules, and although they are sympathetic to her needs on a theoretical level, on a practical basis there is often considerable pressure for her to return to her duties promptly and to assume a full load.

In the face of postpartum blues, decreased energy levels, and new financial stresses, this presents most young marrieds with many added burdens on an already-strained relationship.

Attending-Physician and Faculty Issues

The core of any training program resides in the quality of the supervising physicians and the degree of investment they have in the development and in the careers of their young colleagues. Although many considerations enter into the choice of site for training, including geographic location, subsequent practice opportunities, and family ties, most residents state that the deciding factor was their judgment about the expertise of the faculty and the quality of interaction between supervisors and trainees. In a study at the University of Washington of factors that influenced how medical students and residents rated their clinical teachers, Irby *et al.*[36] stated that the "most noteworthy finding in the present study related to teachers' involvement with trainees. Teachers who were rated as extensively involved with trainees were rated significantly higher in overall teaching effectiveness.... Teacher involvement is probably associated in the trainees' minds as showing a personal interest in them, being concerned about their personal and professional development, and providing appropriate guidance in the clinical setting" (p. 6).

Writing as an intern, Mangione[37] reported that, after three months, she found that her greatest challenges (and also that her level of preparedness was lowest in these areas) were (1) teaching medical students; (2) functioning as an effective ambulatory-care doctor; (3) dealing with the psychosocial issues surrounding terminal illness, death, and dying; and (4) functioning as a cost-conscious member of the medical system. She actually felt quite comfortable performing as a clinician, both in terms of her basic data bank and her expected level of skills in diagnosis and treatment. It was in these former areas where she felt most pressured and least prepared and leaned most heavily on her supervisors for guidance.

Barrows[38] particularly emphasized the growing competitiveness of medicine both for desirable house-officer appointments and for well-paying practice opportunities. He urged that much more attention be paid, both in medical school and during subsequent postgraduate experience, to the exigencies of the medical marketplace.

Patient-Generated Issues

This tends to be a highly subjective area because what disturbs one house officer or challenges his or her capacity to maintain a professional relationship with a given patient is a rather subjective matter. Some residents are very troubled by the intrusive inquiries by parents concerning their child patients; others are not. Some find the argumentative, challenging, and well-informed patients hard to treat, whereas others almost enjoy them. Some are "turned off" by long-term, chronic patients with guarded prognoses, and others find work with this population rewarding.

Nevertheless, there are certain types of patients whom most house officers find very stressful to deal with. When these make up a significant percentage of their case load, there is a tendency to begin to use distancing defense mechanisms in order to cope with the unpleasant and dysphoric feelings they are experiencing. Herzog and his colleagues[39] reported a questionnaire study in which house officers from three different specialties were asked to identify those categories of patients who generated the most unpleasant feelings in them (these might include anger, sadness, anxiety, helplessness, or a general sense of being stressed). There was general agreement that the groups that engendered in them an array of feelings that made it difficult to function as effective clinicians were dying patients or those demonstrating repeated suicide attempts; burn patients; quadriplegics or those with several congenital malformations; sociopathic and dangerous patients; abused children; and those patients who were excessively demanding or communicated a feeling of entitlement.

Career Options and Choices

As noted above, because of the pressures to make decisions early, the need to seek advanced or fellowship appointments if one wishes to subspecialize, and the need to seek out practice opportunities in an increasingly competitive environment, there exists considerable pressure on the young physician to make decisions without knowing all that he or she should know in order to do so wisely. At the same time, they are experiencing the need to master a set of skills and a data base that they consider encompassable and to find something they can be happy with as a professional pursuit for the rest of their lives. This at the age of 24 or 25!

One hundred years ago, Sir William Osler,[40] in his valedictory address entitled "Aequanimitas," spoke to the graduating class of medical students of the University of Pennsylvania in part as follows: "A distressing feature in the life which you are about to enter, a feature which will press hardly upon the finer spirits among you and ruffle their equanimity, is the uncertainty which pertains not alone to our science and art, but to the very hopes and fears which make us men. In seeking absolute truth we aim at the unattainable, and must be content with finding broken portions" (p. 6–7).

Furnham[41] conducted a study of the beliefs of 449 London medical students about nine different specialties. The study demonstrated very clearly how complex career choice must be for the young physician. The author stated "Thus, as nearly all studies have shown, students' attitudes and beliefs are multidimensional and whereas a specialty may be seen as highly positive on one dimension, it may be seen as highly negative on another" (p. 1607).

Meir and Engel[42] conducted a study of 81 physicians, a significant number of whom gave evidence of having made early and perhaps wrong choices about their specialty. By way of interests, they appeared to be mismatched with their careers and yet were spending long days laboring at the care of difficult patients. The implications for quality of care are frightening. Yet, the medical education system drives decision making at juncture points that are not necessarily congruent with the development milestones of the young professional.

In his study of career orientations among interns and residents, Linn[43] stated, "Postgraduate training is experienced in vastly different ways. Furthermore, these differences seem to direct physicians to very different career channels" (pp. 260–261). Linn went on to observe that some young physicians are more "patient-oriented," and that others are more "disease-oriented." In general, these orientations are not recognized in house officers, according to Linn, and are not used as a part of the career counseling that guides them either into more scientific and academic careers or into specialties geared more toward primary patient care.

Depression, Substance Abuse, and Suicide

No discussion of problem areas in postgraduate medical training would be complete without a look at the literature on depression, substance abuse, and suicide. They are lumped together here not because they always occur together, but because they are usually the end points of serious adjustment disorders in house officers that might have been identified earlier but were not. This lack of identification may occur because the individual was so skillful in disguising his or her plight because his or her colleagues were busily covering for him or her, or because the system was insensitive to important signs of maladaptation in one of its key members. There is, of course, a significant body of literature on these areas, and only a few examples can be mentioned here.

Valko and Clayton[44] reported that 53 first-year residents who had just completed an internship reported in interviews that 30% of them had had a depression during their internship year. Four of this group had had suicidal ideation, and three had had a suicidal plan. Of the depressed interns, 31% said that they would not choose medicine again as a career. Most reported that the onset of depression coincided with a heavy increase in work load. In an effort to identify the predictors of depression during the early months of internship, Clark and his colleagues[45] followed 55 first-year residents at a large academic center for one year. Although only 11% of the interns exhibited any psychopathology at the beginning of their training, 40% had experienced at least one major depressive episode, 7% had abused alcohol, and 9% had abused illicit drugs during the year. These percentages are not additive because a few qualified for more than one diagnosis. On a test battery, neuroticism was the only variable that was associated with depression-related work impairment during the first six months. The amount of the work load *per se* did not correlate with depression.

Finally, among the best studies and reviews of substance abuse by medical students and young physicians are the study by McAuliffe[46] and colleagues[46] and that by Stout-Wiegand and Trent.[47] Both of these papers contain very useful bibliographies for the reader who wants more extensive exposure to this area.

ENVIRONMENTAL STRESSES

Financial Problems

It is of particular note that one of the stresses frequently mentioned currently in discussions about house officer experiences is heavy indebtedness resulting from long-term loans required by educational commitments, family, and other obligations. Although this is undoubtedly a very real problem for residents, I was impressed by the absence of literature on this subject and was reminded in my search of how infrequently it came up during the house officer interviews that form the main substance of this book.

Many thoughtful observers have pointed out that an important correlative process occurs with this tendency toward mounting debt in young physicians. That is, medicine may very well once again become a profession for the affluent, as individuals from working-class families and minority groups will be less and less likely to bear this economic burden, which extends well into their productive careers.

Chronic Fatigue and Sleep Deprivation

The matter of chronic fatigue and sleep deprivation is not as straightforward as one might expect. There can be little doubt from many normative studies that, in the average human subject, cognition becomes less efficient, abnormalities in perception and physiological functions may ensue, and there is heightened irritability, self-interest, and a tendency toward labile mood swings. How and whether this reaction impacts on the daily activities of house officers has not been measured in any formal way. We do know that, especially in young, healthy adults, there is remarkable resiliency and a capacity to develop coping mechanisms to deal with fatigue and sleep loss over brief periods of time. As has been illustrated in many of the interviews quoted in this book, a great many house officers do not list chronic fatigue and sleep deprivation among the most important stresses impacting on their daily activities.

Many attending physicians believe that the cost of all the night vigils incurred by young house officers is well worth both the risks and the attendant depletion of energy because it is primarily in this way that they will learn all of the aspects of their patients' illness and will learn the basic philosophy of "attending" to the sick. In fact, most hospitals must walk the fine line between hazing house officers with initiation rites, on one hand, and being sure to provide an intensive enough experience in patient care to season young physicians to the rigors of practice, on the other.[48]

Many who decry the evils of the so-called 36-hour day have few organized data to support their claims of poor patient care beyond anecdotal information from house officers. Several of the interviews in this book would provide equally supportive anecdotal material for the opposing position.

Among the earlier more interesting papers on this subject were two by Friedman and his colleagues[49,50] at Columbia University. In 1971,[49] they administered to sleep-deprived interns an electrocardiographic arrhythmia-detection task and questionnaires assessing mood and subjectively perceived psychophysiological state.

They reported that the subjects were less able to recognize arrhythmias in EKGs when sleep-deprived than in the rested state. Also reported were mood changes and decreased vigor, egotism, and social affection. Many psychophysiological symptoms developed, and a few reported experiencing transient psychopathology. These authors also observed that the "minimum period of deprivation required to produce the changes observed in this investigation was not determined. The threshold for fatigue varies from person to person but it is likely that only a limited amount of sleep loss can be sustained by an intern before emotional and intellectual functioning deteriorates" (p. 203).

In the later paper,[50] the same authors reported that, when interns were sleep-deprived and depressed, they were much less responsive to the demands of patients and staff. There was increased resentment of routine chores and false "emergencies." One intern was quoted as saying, "When I'm tired, like right now, I feel like saying to patients 'let me tell you my problems, don't tell me yours.'"

These same authors further reinforced the speculation that the so-called 36-hour day is not only an initiation rite into an elite society but may also be an outward manifestation of the young physician's wish to become an "iron man," to emulate his or her superiors, and to "possess abilities and powers that transcend what is ordinarily thought of as human" (p. 440).

As late as 1983, Asken and Raham[51] reported finding only six studies in the literature on sleep deprivation and physician performance. These were of limited value because of methodological deficiencies. They concluded that "certainly the research is not what it should be. The general sleep deprivation literature is of questionable applicability, and the physician sleep deprivation literature is undeniably scarce" (p. 387). At a minimum, there exists the requirement of increased time for performance, which may have profound ramifications in emergency or critical care settings.

Yet, these authors quoted an earlier study by Wilkinson and colleagues,[52] who surveyed house officers by asking the question, "Do you think your hours of duty are so long as to impair your ability to work with adequate efficiency?" Of the 2,452 respondents, 3.3% reported "always"; 34% reported "often"; 47.6% reported "occasionally"; 12.2% reported "rarely," and 2.9% reported "never." Although one must be concerned about those who reported impairment, I believe it is also interesting that over 60% of these respondents reported "occasionally" to "never."

Asken and Raham concluded that the stated justifications for night call and sleep deprivation included (1) that sleep-depriving night-call is a valid learning experience; (2) that it is individual idiosyncracies that make night call a negative experience; (3) that night-call schedules do not cause permanent distortions of personal and professional sensitivity in the developing physician and individual; and (4) that quality of care is not compromised by the sleep-deprived physician.

These authors maintained that none of these justifications have been supported by any documentation, and that it is the responsibility of the medical profession and relevant others to engage in scientifically designed studies of these premises or to give them up to common sense.

Finally, Norman Cousins[53] concluded that "the custom of overworking interns has long since outlived its usefulness. It doesn't lead to making better physicians. It is inconsistent with the public interest. It is not really worthy of the tradition of Medicine" (p. 377).

Early Specialization

It is not possible to say too much about the risks of early specialization. Not the least of the problems generated by this trend is the pressure it places on medical students and house officers to make very early judgments about career directions. A more subtle but equally difficult issue is the premature narrowing of the knowledge and skill base of the young physician. Gonnella and Veloski[54] noted that house officers taking Part III of the National Board Examination tended to do better if they were training in a specialty with a relatively broad clinical base (e.g., family practice) than those training in an area with a relatively narrow clinical experience (e.g., pathology). This tends not only to foreclose some aspects of later professional development for the physician, but it makes it very difficult if he or she should decide to change career directions at a later date.

Systems Issues

An entire volume could be written about the many systemic forces that can be brought to bear on the house officer's experience, for better or for worse. These range from the microcosm of the house officer group in which he or she trains to the macrocosm of the overall health-care system of which his or her hospital is a small part. Bates and Carroll,[55] for instance, observed ways in which the hospital administration can ease some of the marital tension for house officers simply by the way in which administrative practices observe the needs of spouses. Jellinek[56] wrote on the recognition and management of discord within house staff teams. In a scholarly presentation, Foreman[57] discussed how changes in the medical care system are impacting on medical education. These are only a few of the dozens of excellent papers available in the literature that address this subject.

CONCLUSION

Although the literature is now beginning to address many important topics in a more careful and well-designed fashion, there is still a shortage of longitudinal research that compares young physicians with matched populations and with normal controls who come from similar socioeconomic backgrounds. Many of the studies are suggestive and helpful, but clearly, we are only at the dawn of truly rigorous research on one of the most critically important segments of our young adult population imaginable.

REFERENCES

1. Puschmann L: A History of Medical Education. London, H.K. Lewis, 1891. (Reprinted by Hafner Publishing Co., New York, 1966.)

2. Flexner A: Medical Education in the United States and Canada, Report to the Carnegie Foundation for the Advancement of Teaching. New York, Carnegie Foundation, 1910.

3. Glaser RJ: The Teaching Hospital and Medical School, in Knowles JH (ed): The Teaching Hospital: Evolution and Contemporary Issues. Cambridge, Harvard University Press, 1966, pp 7–37.

4. AMA Accreditation Council for Graduate Medical Education: 1987–1988 Directory of Graduate Medical Education Programs. Chicago, American Medical Association, 1987, pp VII–VIII, 11–15.

5. Brosin HW: Psychiatry experiments with selection. Social Service Review 22:461–468, 1948.

6. Aldrich CK: The clouded crystal ball: A 35 year follow-up of psychiatrists' predictions. American Journal of Psychiatry 143:45–49, 1986.

7. Becker HS, Geer B: Hughes EC, et al.: Boys in White: Student Culture in Medical School. Chicago, University Press, 1961.

8. Mumford E: Interns: From Students to Physicians. Cambridge, Harvard University Press, 1970.

9. Knowles JH: The Teaching Hospital: Evolution and Contemporary Issues. Cambridge, Harvard University Press, 1966.

10. Coombs RH, Vincent CE: Psychosocial Aspects of Medical Training, Springfield, IL, Charles C Thomas, 1978, pp 429–546.

11. Vaillant GE, Sobowale NC, McArthur C: Some psychological vulnerabilities of physicians. New England Journal of Medicine 287:372–375, 1972.

12. Zabarenko R, Zabarenko L: The Doctor Tree. Pittsburgh, University of Pittsburgh Press, 1978.

13. Small GW: House officer stress syndrome. Psychosomatics 22:860–869, 1981.

14. Loes MW, Scheiber SC: The impaired resident. Arizona Medicine 38:777–779, 1981.

15. Reuben DB: Psychologic effects of residency. Southern Medical Journal 76:380–383, 1983.

16. Ford CV: Emotional distress in internship and residency: A questionnaire study. Psychiatric Medicine 1:143–150, 1983.

17. Winer JA, Ferrono C: Residency training and emotional problems of physicians. Illinois Medical Journal 166:23–26, 1984.

18. Blackwell B, Gutmann MC, Jewell KE: Role adoption in residency training. General Hospital Psychiatry 6:280–288, 1984.

19. Alexander D, Monk JS, Jonas AP: Occupational stress, personal strain and coping among residents and faculty members. Journal of Medical Education 60:830–839, 1985.

20. McCue, JD: Occasional notes: The distress of internship. New England Journal of Medicine 312:449–452, 1985.

21. Hardison JE: Occasional notes: The house officer's changing world. New England Journal of Medicine 314:1713–1715, 1986.

22. Gordon GH, et al.: Stress during internship: A prospective study of mood states. Journal of General Internal Medicine 1:228–231, 1986.

23. Ford CV, Wentz DK: Internship: What is stressful? Southern Medical Journal 79:595–599, 1986.

24. Ziegler JL, Strull WM, Larsen RC, *et al.*: Stress and medical training. Western Journal of Medicine 142:814–819, 1985.
25. Lovett DL: Our new home. JAMA (A Piece of My Mind) 256:3395, 1986.
26. Krell R, Miles JE: Marital therapy of couples in which the husband is a physician. American Journal of Psychotherapy 30:267–275, 1976.
27. Gabbard GO, Menninger RE, Coyne L: Sources of conflict in the medical marriage. American Journal of Psychiatry 144:567–572, 1987.
28. Kelner M, Rosenthal C: Postgraduate medical training, stress and marriage. Canadian Journal of Psychiatry 31:22–24, 1986.
29. Franco K, *et al.*: Conflicts associated with physicians' pregnancies. American Journal of Psychiatry 140:902–904, 1983.
30. Stewart DE, Robinson GE: Combining motherhood with psychiatric training and practice. Canadian Journal of Psychiatry 30:28–34, 1985.
31. Sayers M, *et al.*: Pregnancy during residency. New England Journal of Medicine 314:418–423, 1986.
32. Coombs, RH, Fawz FI: The effect of marital status on stress in medical school. American Journal of Psychiatry 139:1490–1493, 1982.
33. Levy M: Dr. Mom. JAMA (A Piece of My Mind) 257:536, 1987.
34. AMA Ad Hoc Committee on Women Physicians in Organized Medicine: Maternity leave for residents. Report to the Board of Trustees, Chicago, AMA, 1984.
35. American Association of Directors of Psychiatric Residency Training: Report of Task Force on Part Time and Interrupted Training. AADPRT Newsletter, April 1985, pp 34–38.
36. Irby DM, Gillmore GM, Ramsey PG: Factors affecting ratings of clinical teachers by medical students and residents. Journal of Medical Education 62:1–7, 1987.
37. Mangione CM: How medical school did and did not prepare me for graduate medical education. Journal of Medical Education 61:3–10, 1986.
38. Barrows HS: The scope of clinical education. Journal of Medical Education 61:23–33, 1986.
39. Herzog DB, Wyshak G, Stern TA: Patient generated dysphoria in house officers. Journal of Medical Education 69:869–874, 1984.
40. Olser W: Aequanimitas with other addresses. Philadelphia, Blakiston, 1932.
41. Furnham AF: Medical students' beliefs about nine different specialties. British Medical Journal 293:1607–1610, 1986.
42. Meir EI, Engel K: Interests and specialty choice in medicine. Social Science and Medicine 23:527–530, 1986.
43. Linn LS: Career orientations and the quality of working life among medical interns and residents. Social Science and Medicine 15A:259–263, 1981.
44. Valko RJ, Clayton PJ: Depression in the internship. Disorders of the Nervous System 36:26–29, 1975.
45. Clark DC, *et al.*: Predictors of depression during the first six months of internship. American Journal of Psychiatry 141:1095–1098, 1984.
46. McAuliffe WE, *et al.*: Psychoactive drug use by young and future physicians. Journal of Health and Social Behavior 25:34–54, 1984.

47. Stout-Wiegand N, Trent RB: Physicians Drug Use: Availability or Occupational Stress? International Journal of Addictions 16:317–330, 1981.
48. Pye JR: Letter to the editor. American Medical News, American Medical Association, August 28, 1987, p 5.
49. Friedman RC, Bigger TJ, Kornfeld DS: The intern and sleep loss. New England Journal of Medicine 285:201–203, 1971.
50. Friedman RC, Kornfeld DS, Bigger TJ: Psychological problems associated with sleep deprivation in interns. Journal of Medical Education 48:436–441, 1973.
51. Asken MJ, Raham DC: Resident performance and sleep deprivation: A review. Journal of Medical Education 58:382–388, 1983.
52. Wilkinson R, Tyler P, Varey C: Duty hours of young hospital doctors: Effects on the quality of their work. Journal of Occupational Psychology 48:219–229, 1975.
53. Cousins N: Internship: Preparation or hazing. JAMA 245:377, 1981.
54. Gonnella JS. Veloski JJ: The impact of early specialization on the clinical competence of residents. New England Journal of Medicine 306:275–277, 1982.
55. Bates EM, Carroll PJ: Stress in hospitals. The married intern: Vintage 1973. Medical Journal of Austin 2:763–765, 1975.
56. Jellinek M: Recognition and management of discord within house staff teams. JAMA 256:754–755, 1986.
57. Foreman S: The changing medical care system: Some implications for medical education. Journal of Medical Education 61:11–21, 1986.

Part VI

CONCLUSIONS AND RECOMMENDATIONS

Chapter 21

SUMMING UP

Is it reasonable to attempt to draw some conclusions from the experiences of 52 house officers? It may be, if we proceed with caution and if we admit that much of what we think may be speculation. Having surveyed most of the available professional literature, I am reassured, in part, that most studies tend to rely on fewer data than these house officers have supplied. Worse yet, they may draw conclusions based on the experience in one specialty training program. It is even more dangerous to use a sample of impaired house officers, that is, those already referred for some form of clinical intervention.

We originally set out to learn from a random sample of house officers (admittedly, biased by the fact that they were all volunteers) what their experience in training was like, for better or for worse.

Therefore, our interview structure was not aimed at uncovering problems, identifying stresses, or placing blame for failures. On the contrary, we tried to let these physicians tell their stories without leading questions and without introducing our own value system concerning the virtues or evils of postgraduate medical education.

In this sense, perhaps, the information that they supplied may have some genuine, though limited, use.

The advantage in having these house officers tell their stories in a balanced way is that we are not confronted with having to distinguish between "positive" and "negative" stresses, for instance. We know that barring extremes, stress is fundamentally a subjective concept. What is stressful to Peter may not be stressful to Paul.

Furthermore, I have found it troubling to read descriptions of "impaired house officers" or "resident stress syndromes." Sometimes these are a muddle of stress factors (e.g. sleep deprivation), normal developmental tasks (e.g., the transition from studenthood to physicianhood), deficient support systems (e.g., uninterested attendings), and maladaptive outcomes (e.g., substance abuse).

I have not been able to sort out the relationship of these factors to each other, to assign weights to them, or to learn very much from the literature about how they impact on the eventual performance of the physician in practice.

What I did hear these young physicians saying was that, in the midst of the 10-year period between the late teens and the late 20s, a time of struggle, searching, and eventual self-realization for most adults, they had taken on the complicated tasks of becoming medical specialists, and that this process had to occur in what was inevitably a complex and stressful physical and emotional climate.

I came away from these interviews stunned by the awareness of how well most of them seemed to be accomplishing their goals.

DEVELOPMENTAL SEQUENCE OF TRAINING

Like most processes, this one has a beginning, a middle, and an end. The first task of any attending physician, nursing supervisor, or hospital administrator, it seems to me, should be to try to understand the evolution of this process as much as possible. It is in the interest of the clinical department, the hospital, and, most of all, the patient to facilitate this course of events because it should lead to the emergence of competent physicians who give excellent clinical care. Some of the ways in which that might be done are discussed in the next chapter.

First, though, what did these residents tell us about the steps they had to take? Also, what did they tell us about what was accelerating their journey through training and what was impeding it (not the daily carping and complaning, in which all underlings in any large system love to indulge, but what larger, more substantive issues had emerged that extended beyond the boundaries of a single specialty or department)?

There are already some appealing schemas for understanding this developmental process through training. For instance, McGuire[1] made a compelling argument that training not only delays the final achievement of some of the developmental tasks of adolescence, but in some ways, is a recapitulation of the most important aspects of the adolescent experience. Brent[2] conceptualized the training process as one in which the resident faces a series of conflicts (for instance, vulnerability versus omnipotence, activity versus passivity) that must be resolved before there is comfort with being a physician and competence in carrying out the tasks of a specialist.

Certainly, our own house officers inferred that there is considerable basis for these approaches. However, what they also suggested to me, as I have already indicated, was that all real-life educational experiences, like all good mystery novels, have beginnings, middles, and endings.

For me, this is a more useful construct because it is more action-oriented. Attendings and training directors are not always comfortable helping residents with what they view as "adolescent hang-ups," nor are they terribly comfortable with assuming the quasi-psychotherapeutic tasks of conflict resolution.

The so-called beginning has been referred to dozens of times in these interviews in different words, but the kernel of the matter seems to be the painful and frightening shift from 20 years of studenthood to being a responsible physician who takes care of sick people, and is looked to for "orders," for decision making, and for remaining calm, organized, and goal-directed in the face of human pain and catastrophe. The warm cocoon in which the dependent and protected college and medical student lives and works has been stripped away not gradually, but suddenly. I did not stop to count how often terms similar to *cold bath* or *baptism of fire* appeared in these more than 50 interviews, but I would be willing to wager that the total is more than 20.

For those of us who are many years away from the experience, and for those who have never experienced it at all, there may be a lack of appreciation of the depth and intensity of the chain yanking involved.

For some house officers, it lasts through almost the entire year of internship. For others, the transition takes place more rapidly because they are, by nature, rapid adapters and tend to approach new situations in a less guarded and defended way.

Interestingly, many residents stated that they had little trouble with the clinical knowledge and skills they were expected to master during this first year. The crisis they were experiencing had less to do with that kind of mastery and more to do with thinking of themselves as physicians in whom patients could confide and who could be trusted to give competent and timely care.

The "middle" phase of the developmental process seems to be one in which the trainee wants to become an expert. It is time for earning spurs. The mantle of the physician has been donned, and now it must be fortified with the appropriate repertoire of facts and skills. There is a kind of clamoring for responsibility, for new and challenging experiences, for dealing with the most difficult and complicated cases, for being handed the scalpel and the prescription pad and being told, "Go ahead this is your baby. I'm right behind you if you need me."

I would not compare this period to adolescence at all. In fact, residents during this time are more like 9- or 10-year-olds who gobble up new experiences and seem relatively fearless in the face of imminent danger or stress. The medical world is their oyster. They are irritated by the length of training and feel they can master it more quickly. They tend to see their elders as infantalizing them, not trusting them enough with responsibility, and not supporting them to grow up rapidly enough.

In some ways, however, most residents described this as the happiest time of training. The cold bath of internship was behind them, and the real world of practice was in the future. The only item on the agenda was clinical competence. For the resident who might be headed for a life in academic medicine, there was the additional striving for research expertise.

It is during the last year of training that residents begin to struggle with the third step in the developmental process. This involves leaving what has now become, for them, another cocoon (although not nearly as warm and protected as the one they enjoyed as students) and facing the task of building their own professional nest. Questions that they may have confronted only vaguely before now loom large: Is academic life really for me, or do I want the hustle and bustle of private practice? Where should I locate geographically? Do I want to be closer to or further away from my parents? What kind of practice do I really want? Do I want to go solo or be part of a group? What about incorporation? What about hospital appointments and membership in medical societies? What about malpractice insurance? How will I be able to afford an office? How can I stimulate referrals into my practice? Am I really ready to go into practice? Do I need more training? Should I consider a subspecialty? A fellowship?

Those who work with adolescents will already have been asking themselves, "What does he mean that this is not a reiteration of adolescent development? Of course, it is." That is true. But adolescent development itself has been described as a reiteration of the phases of childhood.

Perhaps in too simplified form, I have suggested the outlines of a journey through training as I heard these house officers describe it. For me, this is a useful way to think about the experience because each of these steps suggests ways in which training directors, attendings, and hospital administrators may participate in making the process go more smoothly.

OBSTACLES TO PROFESSIONAL GROWTH

Our house officers took some pains to spell out what they saw as interfering with this adaptive sequence. Certainly, the variety of environmental stresses to which they were subjected during training could impede professional growth. This was especially true if the stresses were unrelieved or extremely intense. As the specific nature of these stresses has just been reviewed in the previous chapter, it would serve no useful purpose to repeat them in this context. Residents may perceive them along a continuum of severity, extending from mere annoyance to paralyzing interference.

Obstacles to professional growth that are more intrapsychic or interpersonal have also been reviewed previously. The most important of these have to do with harboring unrealistic expectations about the magical omnipotent role of physicians in society; conflicts involving relationships with authority figures; and ongoing ambivalence about the choice of medicine or a specialty as a career. In addition, temperamental characteristics that may have been quite useful in achieving success in college and medical school may become self-defeating if they cannot be at least partially modified. So-called Type A behaviors, although often very useful for practicing physicians, may spawn periods of depression in house officers, who are now confronted with their own limitations and no longer able to stay on top of all details, keep a regular schedule, or become comfortable with their inner awareness that work now equals stress.

When work has come to equal stress, in the business of medicine this is easily translated into "Patients equal stress." Resentment may grow in the face of even normal patient demands; this may become exaggerated when such demands are perceived as irrational or excessive.

House officers who are already struggling with their ambivalence about choice of specialty and are now faced with needing to choose a subspecialty in order to secure their financial future may experience yet more resentment and frustration at the demands that the "system" is placing on them.

Life now carries with it the rigorous expectation of managing time with high efficiency, postponing personal gratifications for professional ones, and ordering and reordering priorities for the expenditure of time and energy on a daily basis. Executive functions must find a way to integrate themselves at a higher level of maturity in order to meet these expectations.

INTERNAL COPING MECHANISMS

For any normal young person, this sequence of events is anxiety-producing, to put it mildly. Much of the anxiety can be resolved as time progresses during training and the house officer has an opportunity to look back over his or her track record and to see that he or she is coping. Success breeds success, mastery breeds mastery. Each month, another new clinical rotation handled competently puts an additional notch in the house officer's medical belt.

Although there can be no substitute for this reassurance through experience, other mechanisms help also. The three most common ones that stood out in the interviews of our house officers were denial, depreciation, and projection.

We see the mechanism of *denial* used most frequently to handle the devastating feelings that accompany the responsibility for caring for severely ill or disabled patients or for experiencing the death of a patient. Especially early in training, young physicians transform the patient as person into the patient as disease. For many trainees, the only way to continue to function and care for more patients in the future is to diminish the impact of loss by denying the reality of the feelings associated with it.

By *depreciation*, I am referring to the process by which we are all able to avoid facing the importance of an event or a relationship by belittling it, trivializing it, or making fun of it. The gallows humor of house officers is legend. In 1978, Shem[3] combined the slapstick of *Animal House* with the gritty humor of *M*A*S*H* in his novel about house officer life in a New York hospital (*The House of God*) and introduced the layperson to the world of gomers ("get out of my emergency room," referring to patients who are no longer viewed as human beings), slurpers (attendings who attempt to rise on the academic ladder by licking their way to the top), and blue blazers (hospital administrators whose origin and functions are unknown). In 1987, Konner,[4] in his personal thesis about his journey through medical school entitled *Becoming a Doctor*, extended the macabre glossary further with such *mal mots* as garbageman (referring to a baby born with serious defects), fly sign (describing a patient in terminal condition who lies with his or her mouth wide open, allowing the flies to enter), and crispy critters (children suffering from third-degree burns over most of their bodies), to mention a few. This ability to laugh, often with poorly veiled hostility, at the establishment, at hopeless medical conditions, and at patients who defy their best efforts is an age-old tonic against depression. In these instances, it is carried to extremes but would appear to be dictated by circumstances.

Projection is particularly useful in the face of daily frustration by patients who do not respond, who may not listen, and who do not seem to appreciate. Given the level of self-confidence possessed by even the most competent house officer, it is comforting to be able to share the responsibility for one's failures with insurance companies that insist on discharging patients prematurely, with hospital administrators who know nothing about medicine but are on power trips, and with attending physicians who appear to be on their own ego trips.

All of these mechanisms and more are useful. That is, they help the house officer to survive these difficult periods until the time when his or her self-image is sufficiently secure so that anxiety is decreased and the failures, frustrations, and annoyances of everyday life can be borne without them.

For the occasional house officers whose own experience and track records do not adequately reassure them that they are on the road to a secure professional identity and whose other mechanisms for dealing with their anxiety may not be adequate any longer, there is the inevitable tendency to resort to more pathological devices, such as substance abuse, depression, and even suicide.

There are two rather common manifestations of burn-out that were surprisingly underrepresented in the interviews: chemical abuse and physical illnesses accompanied by frequent work absences. It is not possible to know whether the incidence of these "symptoms" was actually very low in this population, or whether the type of semistructured face-to-face interview used was simply not a very reliable tool for uncovering such data. I can only add that, on the basis of the very detailed day histories collected, these house officers were generally functioning at a very high level of efficiency, considering their respective stages of professional development.

POSITIVE ASPECTS OF STRESS

Lest we leave an erroneous impression, it is important to emphasize that stress is not only a normal, everyday ingredient of living, it usually is a positive force. Most individuals, including physicians, can look back on one or more stressful periods during their lives and affirm the claim that personal growth usually takes place more rapidly and more satisfyingly in the face of resistance. Stockman[5] surveyed a group of 56 pediatric house officers concerning the possible merits of stress. The variety of responses is worth reading in detail, but the most frequent type of reaction was characterized by the two statements, "Stress gives you more self-esteem, knowing you can handle any stressful situation," and "Stress motivates, improves performance (to a point), and keeps you going when tired."

As I reviewed more than 50 interviews that form the basis for this book, I was struck with how infrequently I heard complaints about the stress of training. It seems to me that most of the grumbling was about what were perceived as insensitive administrative policies and attendings who didn't attend.

REFERENCES

1. McGuire T: Developmental Perspective in Stress, in Hoekelman R (ed): Pediatric House Staff Training, Columbus, OH, Ross Laboratories, 1986, pp 14–22.
2. Brent D: The residency as a developmental process. Journal of Medical Education 56:417–422, 1981.
3. Shem S: The House of God. New York, Dell, 1978.
4. Konner M: Becoming a Doctor: A Journey of Invitation into Medical School. New York, Viking, 1987.
5. Stockman J: The Case for Maintaining Stress, in Hoekelman R (ed): Pediatric House Staff Training, Columbus, Ross Laboratories, 1986, pp 52–59.

Chapter 22

SOME WORDS OF ADVICE

In the hope that 35 years as a medical educator and practitioner justifies some privilege in pontificating, I offer the following thoughts. I would hesitate to do so if I thought that the interviews contained in this book did not warrant them. My trepidation is not diminished, however, when I think about the anecdote of the eight-year-old who, when asked who Socrates was, responded, "He was an old man who went around giving advice to everybody. They poisoned him."

Even though I came away from my contacts with these house officers feeling more positive than negative and experiencing a deep sense of admiration of their talents and their tenacity, I continue to harbor some concerns. These are especially important because of their potential impact on patient care.

Some of the problems are societal in origin and require the attention of social institutions, such as the agencies that fund training and pay for clinical care, and of the regulating bodies that license and certify both hospitals and individuals to deliver such care.

Some problems are probably not fixable. High technology is not a fad that will, in time, suffer the fate of the hula hoop and the Cabbage Patch Doll. The continued explosion of our data base in every medical specialty will always threaten to overwhelm both the memory and self-confidence of any young physician.

But I believe that our house officers defined some critical areas where constructive change is possible in our system for training medical specialists as we enter the 1990s, and I think we would do very well to listen, whether we are medical educators, laypeople administering hospitals or other health-care systems, or simply patient-consumers. In all of these roles and others, we have both a global and an individual stake in the manner in which medicine is practiced over the next decades.

Everyone, physicians and laypeople alike, is painfully aware that the cost of medical care is already virtually unbearable. This reality should dictate that whatever solutions we suggest toward making the training of these house officers more functional should not involve increasing that financial burden significantly. My own judgment is that simply throwing money at the kinds of problems described in these interviews would not make them disappear. True, it would be pleasant for house officers to have shorter working hours, higher stipends, and more attendings. In general, these are not realistic suggestions, although some effort is being expended to seek shorter duty periods.

It is axiomatic among the proponents of crisis theory that the comfort and efficiency of the individual will increase if stress is reduced or if supports are increased. With the possible exception of regulations that would eliminate the so-called 36-hour day for interns, there are few if any major interventions that are both feasible and likely to reduce stress.

As I reread all of the interviews that went to make up this book, I continued to be impressed with how few requests there were for stress reduction among the house officers and, conversely, how many direct and indirect pleas there were for altering the ways in which supports were provided.

In addition to a few minor approaches, most of the ways in which this could be accomplished are focused in three areas: (1) educational and training supports; (2) personal and marital supports; and (3) peer supports. The following specific suggestions are concentrated in these areas.

EDUCATIONAL AND TRAINING SUPPORTS

These are by far the highest priority matters. Some involve content areas in which house officer training is being sadly neglected at high cost. Others involve the role of attending physicians and other teachers. The house officers have defined several subjects in which they generally feel unprepared and inadequate to practice properly. Although the following list is not all inclusive, it highlights the topics most commonly mentioned:

1. How does one deal with the patient who seems to be making irrational demands or asking senseless questions? The basic skills necessary to understand how anxiety, confusion, and fear can distort the way in which patients make demands are not taught to most physicians. They do not know how to help the patient ask what is really troubling him or her. Hence, both doctor and patient become increasingly frustrated with each other. Anger and alienation ensue. These skills are not difficult to teach. Most psychiatric residents learn them in the first few months of training. Mastering the skills would make the lives of most young house officers much more bearable, even rewarding.

2. How does one deal with the dying patient? Because there is little assistance in managing their own feelings as they care for the dying patient, young physicians are left to their own resources to cope with the repeated onslaughts of these disturbing emotions. It is inevitable that they become walled off, become denied, or even, through a tortuous process of depreciation, become sources of cavalier joking.

3. On a related matter, it is rare for a house officer to receive any formal training in dealing with disturbed, anxious, or depressed family members. Under the circumstances, they (the family) become sources of added problems, perhaps to be avoided if possible, but rarely to be used as resources in helping the patient. In the process, alienation may occur not only between patient and physician but between physician and all of the significant others in the patient's life.

4. Most training programs prepare house officers only for the clinical side of practice, not the management side. The latter has to do more with learning how to develop an effective system for delivering care in one's office than with learning how to do cost accounting. Because they train in large university-type hospitals, most house officers have little exposure to the microcosm of the office. They have little knowledge of how to recruit, hire, or train their own personnel. There is little awareness of how to create an environment that is conducive to patient comfort, to staff efficiency, and to good clinical care. Yet, they are aware of this deficiency and are troubled by it.

5. The last item in this list is purely an educational issue. It involves the need to arrive at decisions about further training beyond residency so early in the game that such decisions are often based on either erroneous information or, at the least, incomplete information. Considerable thought needs to be given to orienting young physicians to the opportunities for further training, with a particular emphasis on advantages and disadvantages, so that decision making can be less haphazard. A poor choice of subspecialty eventuates in more stress and a physician who feels increasingly trapped by his or her office and patients.

Moving beyond basic content matters in training, our house officers highlighted what sounded to me like several more important concerns. First and foremost among these is the very critical matter of their relationships with their attending physicians. Any hint that the attending may see his or her role as one of hazing house officers leads to immediate resentment. Any poorly disguised variation of this results in the same reaction. For instance, statements like "In my day, we really had it rough as residents; you don't know what hard work is, besides that, we got $50 a month; you people are making a fortune by comparison" or "I don't know why you complain so much; we had a great time as residents; I look back on those days as the happiest of my life. Why are you always bitching?" result in angry looks and sotto voce mutterings.

Most house officers are not looking to be coddled or babied. On the contrary, most are supersensitive to this kind of behavior toward them. What they are seeking are mentors who clearly look on them as investments in the future, as young adults who can be trusted with age-appropriate responsibility. They insist that they will respond to constructive feedback with greater effort, even if it is negative.

Attitudes about the importance of this investment in the house officers, however, must begin at the top. Chairpersons and department heads cannot tell their staff physicians that residents are important people and that teaching is a valuable function in the department and then proceed instead to reward other behavior. Again, economic realities often compel attending physicians to concentrate on bringing in clinical fees and research grants because direct support of training activities from external sources is scarce. But a counterbalancing reality is that these thousands of house officers perform astronomical amounts of service at bargain-basement rates. That, too, is worth a great deal of money in the bottom-line income-and-expense statement of the hospital. In general, these financial hard facts go unrecognized. More likely, hospital administrators will complain about the fact that house officers are receiving high stipends these days. It is rare for them to pause and reconsider what it might cost to deliver the same units of service without the presence of the house officers.

Be this as it may, unless there are clear-cut signs that attendings are rewarded by promotions and by other tangible recognitions for application to teaching and supervising house officers, they cannot be expected to change their current behavior.

This is not a plea to demote clinical service or research. Rather, it is a plea to promote training and education as a coequal. It is unfair for house officers to experience guilt when they request the time and energy of attendings to teach them. In fact, they are not even fully aware of all of the functions for which they need attendings. What they press for is to be taught how to remove a gall bladder safely, to treat hypertension or kidney disease, or to reduce a fracture. What they need equally (and these functions may require more time and energy on the part of an attending) is proper role modeling with respect to dealing with distraught families; handling ethical dilemmas in the resuscitation of terminal patients; experiencing and surviving humility when confronted by diseases that do not behave as they should with treatment; and dealing equitably with hospital administrators, who have their own unavoidable agendas and their own inescapable responsibilities.

House officers are also in sore need of role models who have learned to preserve sufficient control over their personal and professional lives to carry out their tasks within reason. It is not particularly healthy for them to seek identification with models who project an image of superhuman endurance and wisdom. They need attending physicians who can become tired and ask for help; who experience ignorance and seek consultation; who experience anxiety and receive support from colleagues; or who, without guilt or apology, sequester time to share with their families and to pursue personal interests.

Attendings who are sufficiently "attentive" not only to their patients but to their trainees will be alert to the early signs of decompensation or burnout in house officers. These are well described in the literature (see the bibliography at the end of this chapter). This would allow early intervention in the event that special counseling is necessary. It is unlikely that a house officer's peer group will take on the responsibility of reporting these signs to superiors or will feel that it is their responsibility to do so. Anyway, it feels too much like squealing on a school chum and getting him or her into trouble.

Because attending physicians are frequently appearing and disappearing in the lives of house officers as they rotate from service to service, it is vitally important to have one person in the program who has an overview of the house officers. This individual should track or monitor their developmental progression throughout the early, middle, and later phases of training and should consult with the variety of attending physicians who come in contact with each individual. This senior faculty mentor might be the department head in small departments. In larger ones, this probably is not feasible, and the task may require more than one person if there are 40 or 50 residents. Many people believe that this should not be the chief resident (who is basically still also in training) or even the training director, who is, in effect, an administrative officer of the department, and whose basic loyalty must lie with the department rather than with an individual house officer. Furthermore, it is probably important that this person be a kind of generalist who has a broad overview of the specialty rather than a superstar subspecialist who spends every day perfecting his or her skills in one small corner of the specialty.

PERSONAL AND MARITAL SUPPORTS

As many of our trainees indicated, the house officer is rarely neutral about marriage. The spouse is usually seen either as a comfort, a refuge, and a sounding board, or as just one more insatiable demand in a long, hard, merciless day. It is important for training programs to be aware of the family situation in which a house officer is living. There are ways to learn about this personal climate without being intrusive (see the chapter bibliography). For those house officers whose marriages are proving to be stressful, spouse support groups have proved to be helpful in many ways. At a minimum, they provide an understanding and supportive emotional climate in which spouses who may feel neglected and confused can share their own experiences and support each other. At best, each individual in the spouse group may develop insights from more experienced members concerning how to communicate, problem-solve, and maximize the available time with the house officer. The formation and leadership of these groups, once they have been initiated, can be left largely to the spouses themselves, with a small investment of time and energy on the part of a senior social worker in the department.

PEER SUPPORTS

Self-help groups, frequently maligned or burlesqued in the mass media, can have an important place in stress management. Many departments conduct such groups routinely and have reported them to be quite helpful, especially to junior house officers. Obviously, participation in them should be voluntary, their content should be held in confidence, and a more senior person should be available to conduct the groups and ensure that more vulnerable junior members will receive the attention they require. There is a substantial body of literature on this subject. Resources are indicated in the chapter bibliography.

Initial house officer orientations to the department and subsequent, regularly scheduled two- or three-day retreats (to include faculty) have proved to be very useful mechanisms for identifying and mediating stresses. It has become the practice of many hospitals to employ professional management and systems consultants, not only to plan but often to conduct these retreats.

Finally, some medical centers have seen fit to develop special counseling services designed to meet the specific needs of house officers and their families. These really represent interventive rather than preventive services. However, when marital conflict becomes sufficiently severe, or when house officer burnout is imminent, or when questions of chemical abuse are involved, or when a house officer is so troubled by his or her career choice as to become dysfunctional, he or she may require individual and ongoing counseling. The availability of such a service may actually prevent more serious decompensation at a later date, a process that might require termination of training and/or psychiatric intervention.

SUMMARY

In the world of postgraduate medical training, many troubling conditions exist that are plain and simple signs of the times. They are symptomatic of social values, or they are the choppy wake of the ship of scientific progress. If they are fixable, the fixing is probably the responsibility of forces external to the medical profession.

They cannot and should not be used as excuses by the medical establishment to avoid fixing what can be fixed. In the interviews in this book, the consumers of our postgraduate training establishment, the house officers, provided their diagnoses of the ills of the system. In their own pointed and articulate style, they also prescribed many of the treatments. Interestingly, their treatment plan does not involve moving legislative, regulatory, or fiscal mountains. It does not involve shaking the system at its roots or making revolutionary changes in the format of training.

What it does call for is much more thoughtful and organized attention to the deleterious impact of several kinds of stresses on the professional development of the physician—and the introduction of responsible senior physicians and hospital administrators to assist house officers in developing their own strengths to cope with these stresses now and throughout their professional lives.

REFERENCES

American Medical Association: Push to restrict resident's hours gaining momentum. American Medical News, Dec. 4, 1987, pp 6–7.
Blair JP, Greenspan BK: Teams: Teamwork training for interns, residents, and nurses. Hospital and Community Psychiatry 37:633–635, 1986.
Bates EM, Hinton J: Unhappiness and discontent: A study of junior resident medical officers. Medical Journal of Australia 2:606–612, 1973.
Berg JK, Garrard J: Psychosocial support in residency training programs. Journal of Medical Education 55:851–857, 1980.
Bergman AS: Marital stress and medical training: An experience with a support group for medical house staff wives. Pediatrics 65:944–947, 1980.
Borenstein DB: Should physician training centers offer formal psychiatric assis-

tance to house officers? A report on the major findings of a prototype program. American Journal of Psychiatry 142:1053–1057, 1985.

Clark DC, Salazar-Grueso E, Grabler P, et al.: Predictors of depression during the first 6 months of internship. American Journal of Psychiatry 141:1095–1098, 1984.

Doughty R: Strategies for reducing stress: Orientation and retreats in stress, in Hoekelman R (ed): Stress in Pediatric House Staff Training. Columbus, Ross Laboratories, 1986, pp 116–129.

Green M: Individual and group support systems, in Hoekelman R (ed): Stress in Pediatric House Staff Training. Columbus, Ross Laboratories, 1986, pp 146–149.

Howell J, Schroeder D: Physician Stress: A Handbook for Coping. Baltimore, University Park Press, 1984, pp 85–100.

Howell JD, Lurie N, Woolliscroft JO: Worlds apart: Some thoughts to be delivered to house officers on the first day of clinic. JAMA 258:502–503, 1987.

Kahn NB, Schaeffer H: A process group approach to stress reduction and personal growth in a family practice residency program. Journal of Family Practice 12:1043–1047, 1981.

Kanas N, Ziegler JL: Group climate in a stress discussion group for medical interns. GROUP 8:35–38, 1984.

Lefcourt HM, Martin RA, Saleh WE: Locus of control and social support: Interactive moderations of stress. Journal of Personality and Social Psychology 47:378–389, 1984.

New York State Department of Health, Ad Hoc Committee on Emergency Services (Chair, Bell B) 1987, p 4.

Report of New York State Commission on Graduate Medical Education, New York State Department of Health, 1986, pp 37–46.

Reuben DB, Novack DH, Wachtel TJ, et al.: A comprehensive support system for reducing house staff distress. Psychosomatics 25:815–820, 1984.

Siegel B: Enriching personal and professional development: The experience of a support group for interns. Journal of Medical Education 53:908–914, 1978.

Weinstein HM: A committee on well-being of medical students and house staff. Journal of Medical Education 58:373–381, 1983.

Ziegler JL, Kanas N, Strull WM, et al.: A stress discussion group for medical interns. Journal of Medical Education 59:205–207, 1984.

AFTERWORD

The knowledge base of biomedical science has grown rapidly in the last half-century, propelled largely by advances in physics and biology. Although the United States began that period as a solid but relatively minor player on the international medical front, it has now risen to become the undisputed world leader in health care technology. The changes we have witnessed over the past few decades are only the teaser for twenty-first-century medicine. Gamma knives, lasers, and lithotripters are preliminary examples of what will follow. Molecular biology is rapidly infusing every area of medicine. The human genome is about to be mapped, and although gene therapy may be years away, the increasing availability of molecular probes and monoclonal antibodies is completely revamping the way we think about the etiology and pathogenesis of illnesses and is giving us new tools for diagnosis and treatment. Yesterday's miracles, such as x-ray technology, are like pinhole cameras compared to their latter-day replacements, such as the positron emission tomography scanners and magnetic resonance systems that allow us to make dynamic assessments of the functional integrity of organ systems and to monitor vital metabolic processes.

The causes for the spectacular ascent of American medicine are many. It may well have begun with the publication of the Flexner Report in 1910. This seminal investigation of the state of medical schools, commissioned by Andrew Carnegie and conducted by Abraham Flexner, sharply criticized the quality of physician training in the United States and Canada and prompted private foundations and state governments to provide increased financial support to raise the standards of North American medical education. The resulting improvement in the quality of academic programs set the stage for the next leap, the creation of the National Institutes of Health in 1940, which led to generous and stable support for medical education, research, and training in the ensuing decades. Finally, and without any real planning, academic health centers sprang up. By linking medical and other health science schools to teaching hospitals, this new breed of organizational structure provided a nurturing ecosystem for what is today the premier site for postgraduate medical training.

The marriage between universities and teaching hospitals has been exceptionally beneficial for biomedical science, but it has also produced wrenching changes in medical practice. The shift toward specialty and subspecialty training, necessitated by the knowledge explosion and the unceasing introduction of sophisticated new technologies, has gradually changed not only the mission of teaching hospitals but also the relationship between doctors and patients. Most of the hospitals are no longer general facilities but high-tech tertiary-care centers dedicated to the needs of the most seriously ill. Cost-containment efforts imposed by the federal government and other third-party payers have given additional impetus to this shift by narrowing criteria for hospital admission and sharply limiting lengths of stay. As a result, the pace of activities, which was hardly leisurely even a generation or two ago, is fast approaching breakneck speed. Physicians, including postgraduate trainees, have had to learn efficient time-management skills to get patients in and out of the hospitals in hours or days rather than weeks or months. The rise in medical malpractice suits has imposed the additional burden of documenting all activities, including every discourse between doctor, patient, and family. In short, the strong, solid image of yesterday's physician in charge has become a haze in the hospital hall. No longer does each patient have a single doctor. More often than not, the patient's condition requires consultation from one or more subspecialists, all of whom have contact with the patient and occasionally assume overall responsibility for care. Furthermore, the modern hospital environment includes a host of highly trained technicians whose task is to operate the intricate new machinery for monitoring vital systems and who thus spend more time with the patient than the doctors do. More often than not, however, none of these very busy health care professionals has the time or the preparation to explain the modern medical system to the patient.

Thus, whereas this new-age care may be better in the technical sense of quicker cures and decreased mortality, patients and their families today do not feel better cared for than they did in previous generations. They have difficulty understanding the complexity of diagnostic and treatment procedures, particularly when they have to decide, often under the pressure of time, whether they should authorize the use of heroic measures to prolong life without knowing if the additional burden will yield the hoped-for benefit. Under these circumstances, even the most careful explanation of choices tends to heighten anxiety, rather than allay it, causing both patients and families to forget what they were told. While they may have an intellectual appreciation of the time constraints under which physicians operate, they want someone to take the time to comfort them. The perceived lack of caring may make them belligerent, hostile, or threatening, further undermining the already tenuous doctor–patient relationship.

Whereas medical practice has undergone a fundamental transformation, medical education is still grounded in its post-Flexnerian traditions. Although electronic textbooks are gradually replacing the printed format to facilitate continuous updating, medical students are still taught as though almost everything that is known can be committed to memory. Postgraduate education, too, contains many of the original ingredients of the German teaching hospital model. To be sure, the process has been formalized over the years and the period required to complete special training extended. However, contrary to the approach in other postgraduate academic programs in the United States, interns and residents tend to be treated like students, not junior colleagues.

Reforms have been slow and limited. Although house staff are literally frontline soldiers, they are almost never asked by hospital administration to identify problems or assist in finding solutions. Interns and residents continue to function in a social system in which everyone, including patients, has well-defined rights while they have mostly responsibilities. That they can be dressed down and criticized publicly like naughty schoolchildren is not without its consequences on their relationships with patients and other health professionals.

In recent years, medical schools, recognizing that students are preselected on the basis of their quantitative rather than their social skills, have introduced courses to enhance their appreciation of the intricacies and fragility of the doctor–patient relationship and to sensitize them to the many ethical issues involved in diagnostic and treatment decisions. It is understandable that these well-meaning efforts have not achieved their stated purpose, for the autocratic nature of the attending's relationship to the house staff does more to obliterate than to reinforce values we hold dear—at least in principle.

Given this context, Dr. Cohen has presented with elegant simplicity the issues that need to be addressed, and his book should be on the reading list of all of us who have responsibility for postgraduate training. To his credit, he took great care to stay within the limits of the data obtained from interviews with his young colleagues. The interns and residents believe that postgraduate training needs to be fine-tuned but that massive changes are not necessary. Maybe they are right, but I am inclined to be a harsher critic. My own view is that we need to be jolted out of our complacency. The Flexner Report did for 1920s American medicine what Sputnik did for 1950s physics and engineering science: Both caused considerable embarrassment, but out of that embarrassment grew something exciting and better. Postgraduate medical training of the 1990s would benefit from a similar remedy.

Thomas Detre, M.D.
Senior Vice President
Health Sciences
University of Pittsburgh

GLOSSARY

Acoustic neuroma   A progressively growing, benign tumor within the canal that carries the nerve that transmits impulses between the ear and the brain; as it grows it may cause pressure on the nerve, resulting in deafness, pain, dizziness, and other symptoms.

Adhesion   A band of tissue that causes two body structures to adhere to each other abnormally.

Airway   The route by which air passes into and out of the lungs, or a device for ensuring such unobstructed passage, usually used during anesthesia.

Ambulatory   Able to walk; in medicine, refers primarily to services and patients who can be served as outpatients and, therefore, who do not need admission to the inpatient units of the hospital.

Anal sphincter   The band of muscle fibers that constricts the external opening of the rectum and that, when relaxed, permits defecation.

Anaphylactic   Referring to an extreme allergic reaction; may threaten the patient's life, especially if membranes lining the airway swell sufficiently to cause strangulation.

Anastomosis   A connection or communication between two vessels or body spaces either by surgery or by natural causes.

Aneurism   A bubble or sac formed by the thinning of the wall of a blood vessel. This not only produces an abnormal swelling, but because of the stretching of the vessel wall, there is danger of rupture and subsequent hemorrhage into the surrounding tissues.

Angina   Unless otherwise specified, a sharp, suffocating pain in the chest usually caused by a decrease in oxygen supply to the heart muscle.

Angiogram   An X ray of one or more blood vessels, which are filled with an opaque dye to make them stand out.

Anticonvulsive agent   A type of medication taken for the purpose of preventing epileptic seizures.

Arteriovenous malformation   A congenital defect resulting in an abnormal connection between an artery and a vein.

Arthroscopy   Examination of the interior of a joint by using an instrument; arthroscopic surgery involves operating on a joint while viewing it through this instrument without having to make a large incision and lay open the entire joint.

Atrial fibrillation   Rapid, random contraction of the muscles of one of the smaller chambers of the heart, causing an irregular heart beat.

Attending   In medical practice, refers to the physician who has primary responsibility for the patient's diagnosis and treatment. Certain aspects of care may be delegated to nurses, house staff, or others, but the "attending" physician remains the accountable physician.

Autism or early infantile autism   A condition of childhood characterized by the presence of many stereotyped behaviors and an inability to relate to others in the usual way or to use verbal language for communication.

Botryoid sarcoma   A rare form of malignant tumor in which the external structure resembles a bunch of grapes.

Cardiac catheterization   Passage of a small tube or catheter through a vein in the arm or the leg and into the heart for the purpose of diagnosing a variety of heart diseases.

Carotid artery   The major artery that runs through the neck and supplies blood to the head structures and the brain.

Cerebrospinal fluid   The fluid contained in the ventricles of the brain and the central canal of the spinal cord.

Cervical vertebra   One of the bones (located in the neck region) of the spinal column, which contains and protects the spinal cord.

Clerkship   The practical clinical experience that medical students receive with patients under the close supervision of a teaching physician. This apprenticeship period follows at least two years of laboratory and theoretical study and is accompanied by lectures on subjects pertaining to illnesses and patient care.

Cochlear implant   Surgical replacement of the spiral structure of the inner ear.

Colostomy   An operation used to create an artificial opening between the large intestine and the surface of the body, usually necessary when the bowel between the point of the opening and the rectum is blocked or is not functioning.

Continuity clinic   An outpatient service where patients who require ongoing care are assigned to one physician, who then may maintain constant contact, may become familiar with them, and may provide individualized care.

Coumadin   A drug that reduces the risk of blood clotting; frequently also used in rat poison.

CT scan   Abbreviation for computerized tomography scanning, a procedure in which emerging X rays are measured by a scintillation counter, and its impulses are recorded on a magnetic disc and then, by use of a computer, displayed as a cross section of the body part being studied.

Cytology   The study of the structure and function of body cells both in the normal and the disease states.

Ectopic pregnancy   A pregnancy occurring elsewhere than in the normal place in the uterus, usually in one of the Fallopian tubes leading from the ovary to the uterus.

Electrocardiogram   A tracing showing the electrical activity as the heart muscle is stimulated to function by the nerve supply of the heart.

Endoscopy   Inspection of a body organ by means of a device designed to permit direct visual access without requiring surgical invasion of the space.

ENT   The specialty of medicine that is concerned with diseases of the ear, nose, and throat (otolaryngology).

Epiglossitis   Inflammation of the lidlike covering over the larynx (voice box), which prevents fluids and food from entering the breathing passages during swallowing.

ER   Abbreviation for *emergency room*; the location in most hospitals where patients are first seen by the nurse and doctor, whether or not their complaint is of an emergency nature.

Fellow   In medical education, usually denotes a physician who has completed a residency in one of the specialty areas and is now taking advanced training in a subspecialty (for instance, pediatric cardiology following pediatrics).

Flat plate   An X ray taken through one plane of the body.

Fluoroscope   A device for examining deep structures of the body and projecting the pictures on a fluorescent screen.

Gastroenterologist   A physician specializing in the medical (versus surgical) management of the organs of digestion and elimination (mouth, esophagus, stomach, small and large intestine, liver, and gall bladder).

Gross specimen   A specimen of tissue or an entire body part that can be examined, measured, and described by observation by the naked eye, in contrast to a microscopic specimen.

H. and P.   History and physical examination.

Hemodynamics   The study of the manner in which blood moves through the body and of the forces that influence this movement.

Hepatic artery   The vessel that carries the major blood supply to the liver.

House officer and house staff   The derivation of this term is not completely clear, though the word *house* here probably refers to the hospital; technically, any physician in training as an intern, a resident, or a fellow.

Hypotension   Abnormally low blood pressure.

Hypovolemia   An abnormally low volume of circulating blood plasma in the body.

ICU   Abbreviation for *intensive care unit*, a hospital unit that provides specialized personnel and equipment for the care of seriously ill patients who require immediate and continuous attention.

Indwelling catheter   A catheter that is held in position for extended periods.

Inguinal hernia   Protrusion of a portion of an organ, usually a loop of bowel, through the inguinal canal in the groin area of the body.

Inhalation anesthesia   Anesthesia that is breathed in by the patient in contrast to anesthesia that is injected or applied to the surface of the body.

Intern   A graduate physician who is usually practicing during his or her first year following graduation from medical school and who is not licensed to care for patients independently but only under the direct supervision of another physician who is licensed. Most internships are for one year and may be in a single specialty, like internal medicine or surgery, or they may be mixed, with several specialties being represented. Policies regulating internships are determined by each state, as are laws governing medical licensure. An intern is a member of the house staff and may be referred to as a house officer.

Intubate   To insert a tube, usually through the larynx or voice box, in order to ensure the unobstructed passage of air (or anesthesia during surgery).

Laryngectomy   Surgical removal of the larynx, or voice box.

Magnetic resonance imaging   A diagnostic device for taking pictures of body parts by exposure of the patient to radio waves while he or she is positioned in a powerful magnetic field.

Malignant cardiac rhythm   A pattern of heart beats that denotes that the heart is pumping blood in an abnormal way.

Maxillofacial   Referring to the portion of the bony structure of the face that forms the upper jaw, the palate, the nasal cavity, and the floor of the socket containing the eye.

Metastatic carcinoma   A malignant tumor that spreads (usually through the blood stream) to other parts of the body.

Microvascular surgery   Extremely fine surgery involving the smallest blood vessels of the body.

Myasthenia gravis   A disease characterized by fatigue, exhaustion of muscles, and progressive paralysis. Muscles of the face and neck are most commonly affected.

Neuroma   A tumor that grows from cells of the nervous system.

Neurotic   A term no longer in fashion in psychiatry but generally referring to a person suffering from a disorder characterized by severe anxiety caused by unresolved inner conflicts.

Nuclear medicine   The specialty of medicine concerned with the use of radionuclides for diagnosis and treatment.

OB or OB/GYN   Abbreviation for *obstetrics* or *obstetrics and gynecology.* The medical specialty concerned with the care of pregnant women, childbirth, and the disorders common to the female pelvic region.

Oncology   The medical specialty concerned with the study, diagnosis, and treatment of tumors.

Opthalmology   The specialty of medicine concerned with diseases of the eye and the surrounding tissues.

Optometry   Measurement of the accuracy of vision and the use of lenses to correct visual difficulties.

OR   Abbreviation for *operating room.*

Otitis media   Inflammation of the middle ear.

Otolaryngology   The specialty of medicine that is concerned with diseases of the ear, nose, and throat (ENT).

Pericarditis   Inflammation of the fibrous membrane that covers the heart.

Peritoneum or peritoneal space   The peritoneum is the membrane that covers the organs in the abdominal cavity. The space between this membrane and the inner wall of the abdomen is the peritoneal space.

Plasmapheresis   A process of removing blood, separating the cells from the plasma, and returning the cells suspended in a proper solution; method useful either for obtaining normal plasma or for treating certain diseases of the blood.

Port wine hemagioma   A congenital malformation in which many small, closely packed blood vessels form a mass usually close to the surface of the skin. Because of the concentration of blood in the area, the color of the mass has been called *port wine.*

Preeclampsia   A toxic condition of late pregnancy characterized by high blood pressure, abnormal amounts of protein excreted in the urine, and a swelling of body parts because of fluid retention.

Psoriasis   A chronic, recurrent skin rash that has a red base and is covered by white scales; most commonly appears on the scalp, the arms, and the legs.

Psychopathology   Mental and emotional disorders.

Psychophysiological   Most commonly refers to the presence of bodily symptoms caused by or associated with mental or emotional factors.

Psychosocial   Having to do with both psychic and social aspects.

Psychotherapy   Treatment carried out by mental and interpersonal means in contrast to physical or biological agents; might include suggestion, hypnosis, abreaction, psychoanalysis, behavior modification, and others.

Pulmonary edema   Abnormal retention of fluid in the lungs causing difficulty in breathing.

Pulmonary embolus   A clot carried by the blood stream from another part of the body to one of the blood vessels of the lung, causing blockage of flow and usually, therefore, death of the surrounding lung tissue.

Pulmonary lobectomy   Surgical removal of one lobe of the lung.

Renal colic   Acute abdominal pain caused by a problem in the kidney, most often the passage of a kidney stone.

Resident   A resident is a physician who has completed an internship and is now in the process of training in one of the medical specialties. In most states, residents are licensed physicians. The usual length of a residency is three years, although some may be longer. A resident is a member of the house staff and may be referred to as a house officer.

Retractor   An instrument for maintaining exposure during surgery by separating the edges of a wound and holding back the underlying structures.

Rheumatic heart disease   Involvement of the tissues of the heart as a sequel to rheumatic fever.

Rounds   A review of the status of each inpatient currently on a hospital unit by the house staff and the attending physician. May be either "walking rounds," in which each patient is visited and examined, or "chart rounds," during which patient status is monitored by a review of each chart.

Serum amylase   A substance produced primarily in the pancreas and used by the body in the digestion of starch. It appears in the blood stream normally and is a sensitive indicator of damage occurring to body organs, especially the pancreas, the liver, the kidney, and the gall bladder.

T and A   Abbreviation for *tonsillectomy and adenoidectomy,* a surgical procedure by which the tonsils and adenoids are removed.

Tarry stools   Stools containing large amounts of blood that has turned black because of the action of the body's digestive substances on it; denotes bleeding somewhere high in the gastrointestinal tract.

Thoracic surgery   Surgery involving the structures of the chest.

Thymus gland   A gland that is located in the front of the upper chest and that plays a role in controlling the body's immune system.

Toxemia   Generally caused by the release of toxic substances from bacteria into the blood stream. When used in connection with pregnancy, the term denotes a group of disorders of metabolism that can interfere with the normal course of pregnancy and may produce convulsions, and even death in the mother.

Tympanectomy   Surgical removal of the membrane (ear drum) that covers the middle ear.

Vagal   Refers to the vagus nerve, which, when highly stimulated, may produce marked flushing of the skin, cramping with pain, constipation, and excessive sweating.

Ventricular fibrillation   Small, local contractions of the muscle fibers of one of the large chambers of the heart. This is an abnormal rhythm or beat that results in inefficient pumping of blood.

Vestibular nerve   The nerve that connects the inner ear to the brain and functions to transmit sensations of balance or equilibrium.

V tach (ventricular tachycardia)   Abnormally high rate of action of one of the two large pumping chambers of the heart.